Scott, Foresman

FITNESS FOR LIFE

Third Edition

Authors

Charles B. Corbin
Professor of Physical Education
Arizona State University
Tempe, Arizona

Ruth Lindsey
Professor Emeritus
 of Physical Education
California State University
Long Beach, California

Editorial Offices: Glenview, Illinois
Regional Offices: Sunnyvale, California
Tucker, Georgia • Glenview, Illinois
Oakland, New Jersey • Dallas, Texas

CONTRIBUTORS

Reviewers and Content Specialists

Phyllis A. Blatz
Executive Director
California Association for Health, Physical
Education, Recreation, and Dance (CAHPERD)
Sacramento, California

Sharon Colacino, Ph.D
Anatomist
Purdys, New York

Lila L. Farr
Physical Education Teacher
Consultant
Ocean View High School
Huntington Beach, California

Isabelle D. Holston
Chairman, Physical Education Department
Teacher/Coach
Physical Education Curriculum Committee Member
DeKalb County School System
Decatur, Georgia

Michael J. Schaffer
Supervisor of Health Education
Prince George's County Public Schools
Upper Marlboro, Maryland

Dorothy A. Starbird
Evans High School
Orlando, Florida

Medical Consultant

Dr. Jeffrey L. Boone, M.D.
Medical Director
Institute of Stress Medicine
Porter Memorial Hospital
Denver, Colorado

Adapted Physical Education Consultant

Dr. Frank Short
Department of Physical Education and Sport
State University of New York
Brockport, New York

ISBN: 0–673–29749–7 (Hardcover)
ISBN: 0–673–29750–0 (Softcover)
Copyright © 1990, 1993
Scott, Foresman and Company, Glenview, Illinois
All rights reserved.
Printed in the United States of America.

345678910KPK999897969594

CONTENTS

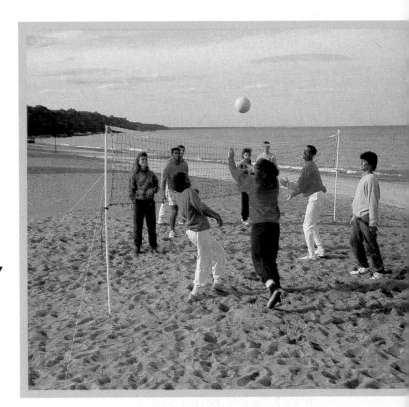

16

FITNESS AND SPORTS 196

17

PLANNING YOUR EXERCISE PROGRAM 204

18

FITNESS AND YOUR FUTURE 214

1

FITNESS FOR ALL

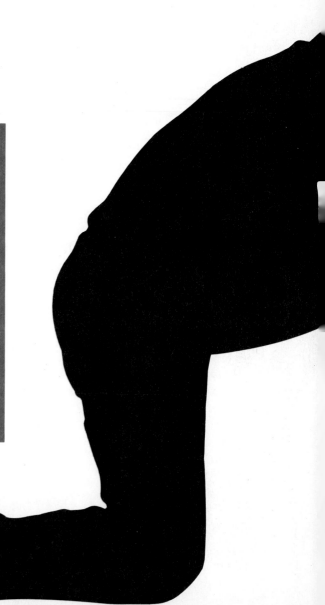

CHAPTER OBJECTIVES

After reading this chapter, you should be able to:

✔ Define total fitness.

✔ List benefits of regular exercise.

✔ Name and discuss the five parts of health-related fitness.

✔ Name and discuss the six parts of skill-related fitness.

✔ Discuss reasons why people do or do not exercise regularly.

Most people realize the value of being active and fit, no matter what their age. Still, the teenage years and the young-adult years are the times in a person's life when fitness can improve more quickly than at any other times. In this chapter, you will learn about the advantages of regular exercise. You will also learn about the parts of health-related physical fitness and skill-related physical fitness.

TOTAL FITNESS

The term "fitness" implies more than just physical fitness and exercise. Everyone should try to achieve *total fitness*—fitness of the whole person including physical, mental, social, and emotional fitness. Good nutrition, good dental health, and ample relaxation and sleep are important to total fitness. A totally fit person is in good physical condition and is socially and emotionally mature for his or her age.

Each area of total fitness depends on, and is related to, the others. For example, the success of a physical fitness program depends not only on your physical abilities, but also on your mental attitude about the program, your patience with your body's response to the program, and other factors. As you learn about physical fitness, note how it ties into total fitness and, most importantly, how it can improve *your* total fitness.

PHYSICAL FITNESS

Physical fitness is the ability of your body systems, including your muscles, skeleton, and heart, to work together efficiently. Being efficient means being able to do the most physical activity with the least amount of effort.

If you are physically fit, you will be able to enthusiastically participate in school and recreational activities. Being fit and active makes both work and recreation more enjoyable. Developing and maintaining physical fitness requires considerable effort, but the results are well worth it. Of course, physical fitness alone will not make you a happy, well-adjusted person. However, without physical fitness, you will have less energy to enjoy life.

HAVE YOU HEARD?

The United States Government has established nationwide health goals, to be met by the year 2000, in a report entitled *Healthy People 2000*. One of the primary goals is to increase the physical activity levels of American citizens, many of whom are inactive.

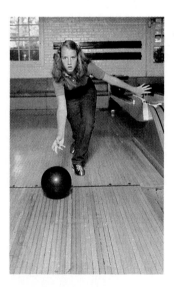

Exercise helps people feel better in general.

BENEFITS OF PHYSICAL FITNESS

Listed below are some benefits you might notice if you follow a regular program of physical activity.

BE HEALTHY In a recent survey, a group of adults were asked to choose one thing they thought would make them happy. They usually said "good health." When a group of young people were asked the same question, they were less likely to be concerned about good health than older people. However, showing concern for your health when you are young plays a vital role in good health later in life.

Regular exercise is essential to good health. If you are active and fit, you are less likely to suffer from heart disease, backache, or obesity. Health experts also believe that regular exercise can lower the risk of high blood pressure, ulcers, and even some forms of cancer.

FEEL GOOD Good health is more than freedom from illness or disease. Studies show that people who exercise regularly "feel good about life." Like the person shown here, they believe that fitness and exercise help them to work better, and to resist fatigue, illness, and injuries. These people also report that they sleep better and feel better in general.

LOOK GOOD Most people are concerned with the way they look. In fact, one study shows that 94 percent of all men and 99 percent of all women would change some part of their personal appearance if they could. People are most concerned with their weight (weighing too much or too little), the size of their waists and thighs, their muscles, hair, and teeth. Being fit and active can give you some control over some of these features and help you look your best. Many physical characteristics, such as bone size and height, are determined by *heredity*— the passing of genetic traits from parents to children. However, a regular fitness program can help you build muscle, control body fat, and improve posture, regardless of heredity.

In social settings, such as dating, meeting new people, and interviewing for jobs, first impressions are often important. For example, a slumped, slouched-over look might keep you from being hired for a job. Working to look your best can help you feel confident and good about yourself. These feelings show themselves to others.

ENJOY LIFE If you are physically fit, you will find that activity is a great way to spend free time. Some people prefer outdoor sports, such as tennis and soccer. Others like indoor sports, such as handball and bowling. Some people like the competitive nature of softball and basketball. Still others prefer such noncompetitive activities as bicycling and hiking. Thanks to a wide choice of activities, you should be able to find an activity that you enjoy and that helps you stay fit.

HEALTH-RELATED PHYSICAL FITNESS

Physical fitness is made up of eleven parts; five parts are health-related, six parts are skill-related. As the names imply, *health-related fitness* helps you stay healthy, while *skill-related fitness* helps you perform well in sports and activities that require certain skills. The five parts of health-related physical fitness are described below. Each will be fully discussed in later chapters.

● *Cardiovascular fitness* is the ability to exercise your entire body for long periods of time. Cardiovascular fitness requires a strong heart, healthy lungs, and clear blood vessels to supply your body with oxygen.

● *Strength* is the amount of force your muscles can produce. Strength is often measured by how much weight you can lift. People with good strength can perform daily tasks efficiently, that is, with the least amount of effort.

● *Muscular endurance* is the ability to use your muscles many times without tiring. People with good muscular endurance are likely to have better posture and fewer back problems. They are also better able to resist fatigue than people who lack good muscular endurance.

● *Flexibility* is the ability to use your joints fully—through a wide range of motion. You are flexible when your muscles are long enough and your joints are free enough to allow movement. People with good flexibility have fewer sore or injured muscles.

● *Body fatness* is the percentage of body weight that is fat when compared to other tissue, such as bone and muscle. For example, a person who weighs 120 pounds of which 24 pounds is fat has a body fatness of 20 percent. People who are in the proper range of body fatness are more likely to avoid illness and even have lower death rates than those outside these ranges. The extreme ranges are the most dangerous; too little body fat, like too much, can cause health problems.

To be healthy, you should have at least some of each of the health-related parts of fitness. If you do, you are less likely to develop a hypokinetic condition—a health problem caused partly by lack of exercise. Examples include heart disease, high blood pressure, backache, stomach ulcer, and being overfat. You will learn more about hypokinetic conditions in Chapter 5.

People who are fit feel better, look better, and have more energy. You do not have to be a great athlete to have good health and feel fit. Regular exercise can improve anyone's health-related fitness.

HAVE YOU HEARD?

Most people believe that physical activity is important, but only about 60 percent say that they exercise regularly. Only about one-third of these people are exercising enough to be fit.

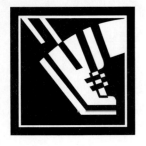

ACTIVITY

HEALTH-RELATED PHYSICAL FITNESS

WORKSHEET 1-1

Use worksheet 1-1 to record your results of this activity.

Use this activity to get a better understanding of the parts of health-related physical fitness. The activities are not intended to test your fitness; future self-evaluations will do so. Remember to warm up before and cool down afterwards.

RUN IN PLACE

- This activity focuses on your cardiovascular fitness.
1. Find your pulse.
2. Run 120 steps in the same place for 1 minute. A step is every time a foot hits the floor.
3. Rest for 1 minute. Count your heart rate for 30 seconds. See if it is 75 or lower.

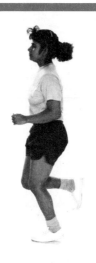

TWO-HAND ANKLE GRAB

- This activity focuses on flexibility.
1. With heels together, bend forward and reach with your hands between your legs and behind your ankles.
2. Clasp your hands in front of your ankles.
3. Interlock your hands for the full length of your fingers. You must keep your feet still.
4. Hold for 5 seconds.

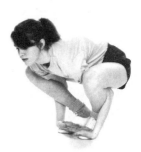

SINGLE LEG RAISE

- This activity focuses on muscular endurance.
1. Position your upper body on a table so your feet touch the floor. Extend one leg straight out.

2. Complete up to 25 leg raises. You can use an ankle weight to make this activity more difficult.

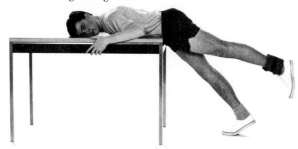

ARM PINCH

- This activity focuses on body fatness.
1. Let your right arm hang relaxed at your side. Have a partner pinch the skin and fat under the skin on the back of your arm. Pinch halfway between your elbow and shoulder.
2. Have your partner use a ruler to measure the skin thickness. If you are a male is your thickness no greater

than 5/8 of an inch? If you are a female, is your thickness no greater than 7/8 of an inch?

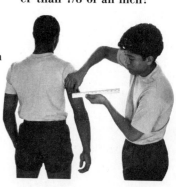

HALF PUSH-UP

- This activity focuses on strength. See page 80 for directions for this exercise.
1. Males do 3.
2. Females do 1.

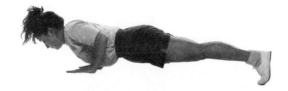

SKILL-RELATED PHYSICAL FITNESS

Of the eleven parts of physical fitness, six parts are considered skill-related. Each skill-related part is described below, but will be discussed more fully in later chapters.

- *Agility* is the ability to change the position of your body quickly and to control your body's movements. People with good agility are likely to be good at activities such as wrestling, diving, and soccer.
- *Balance* is the ability to keep an upright posture while standing still or moving. People with good balance are likely to be good in activities such as gymnastics and ice skating.
- *Coordination* is the ability to use your senses together with your body parts, or to use two or more body parts together. People with good eye-hand or eye-foot coordination are good at hitting and kicking games such as baseball, tennis, soccer, and golf.
- *Power* is the ability to use strength quickly. It involves both strength and speed. People with good power might have the ability to put the shot, throw the discus, high jump, play football, and speed swim.
- *Reaction time* is the amount of time it takes you to move once you realize the need to act. People with good reaction time are able to make fast starts in track or swimming, or to dodge a fast attack in fencing or karate. Good reaction time is necessary for your own safety while driving or walking.
- *Speed* is the ability to perform a movement or cover a distance in a short period of time. People with leg speed can run fast, while people with good arm speed can throw fast or hit a ball that is thrown fast.

Different sports require different parts of skill-related fitness. Most sports require several of these parts. If you are good at these skill-related parts of fitness, you might be good at various sports and games. If not, you can improve your abilities in these areas with practice.

Some people have more natural ability in skill areas than others. No matter how you score on the skill-related parts of fitness, there is some type of physical activity you can enjoy. Keep in mind that good health does not come from being good in skill-related fitness. Good health comes from doing activities designed to improve your health-related fitness.

ACTIVITY

SKILL-RELATED PHYSICAL FITNESS

WORKSHEET 1-2

Use worksheet 1-2 to record your results of this activity.

Try these activities to get a better understanding of the parts of skill-related physical fitness. The activities are not intended to test your fitness; future self-evaluations will do so. Remember to warm up before and cool down afterwards.

LINE JUMP

• This activity focuses on agility.
1. Balance on your right foot on a line on the ground.
2. Leap onto the left foot so that it lands to the right of the line.
3. Leap across the line onto the right foot; land to the left of the line.
4. Leap onto the left foot, landing on the line.

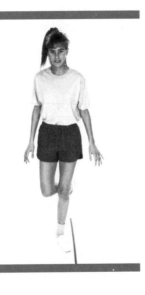

DOUBLE HEEL CLICK

• This activity focuses on speed.
1. Jump into the air and click your heels together twice before you land.
2. Your feet should be at least 3 inches apart when you land.

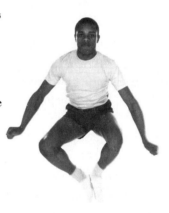

BACKWARD HOP

• This activity focuses on balance.
1. With your eyes closed, hop backward on one foot for 5 hops.
2. After the last hop, hold your balance for 3 seconds.

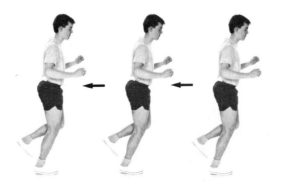

DOUBLE-BALL BOUNCE

• This activity focuses on coordination.
1. Hold a volleyball in each hand. Beginning at the same time with each hand, bounce both balls at the same time, at least knee high.
2. Bounce both balls 3 times in a row without losing control of them.

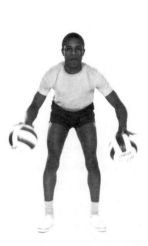

KNEES TO FEET

- This activity focuses on power.
1. Kneel so that your shins and knees are on the mat. Hold your arms back. Point your toes straight backward.
2. Without curling your toes under you or rocking your body backward, swing your arms upward and spring to your feet.
3. Hold your position for 3 seconds after you land.

COIN CATCH

- This activity focuses on reaction time.
1. Point your right elbow in front of you. Your right hand, palm up, should be by your right ear. If you are left-handed, do this activity with your left hand.
2. Place a coin as close to the end of your elbow as possible.
3. Quickly lower your elbow and grab the coin in the air with your right hand before it touches the ground. Drop the coin from your elbow; do not throw it.

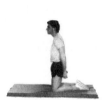 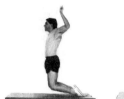 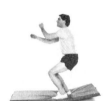 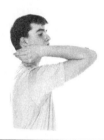 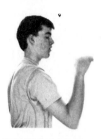

ATTITUDES TOWARD FITNESS AND EXERCISE

Your attitudes toward physical activity help determine whether you will exercise now and throughout your life.

NEGATIVE ATTITUDES Even when they know the importance of exercise, people sometimes make up excuses to not exercise.

- *"I don't have the time. I'm too busy to exercise. "*
Most people have busy schedules. However, people who exercise regularly know that they work more efficiently than if they were inactive.

- *"People might laugh at me."*
Most people do not laugh at others who try their best. Choose an activity you enjoy and stay with it. The more you perform your activity, the more you will improve. The better you will feel about yourself.

- *"I don't want to get all sweaty."*
There is no effortless way to get physically fit. You have to exercise if you want to be fit. Allow more time to clean up after exercise.

- *"I'm already in good condition. I don't need to exercise."*
Use the self-evaluations in this book, and then take an honest look at yourself. Are you as fit as you thought? Exercise can help you get in shape and help you *stay* in shape.

- *"It's hard to get in shape when you haven't exercised regularly."*
Start gradually if you have not exercised regularly. Set realistic goals. Becoming fit takes time and effort.

- *"I was never good at sports. Anyway, sports are for athletes."*
You do not have to be a great athlete to enjoy exercise and sports. Winning is fine, but an activity is more than winning.

HAVE YOU HEARD?

Physical fitness is just as important for disabled people as it is for the able-bodied. In addition, exercise provides greater personal independence for the disabled person.

HAVE YOU HEARD?

The term "runner's high" refers to the feeling of well-being that a person gets from training regularly. Some scientists feel that this good feeling might come from chemical changes in the brain.

POSITIVE ATTITUDES You can develop positive attitudes about exercise. Listed below are some reasons people like to exercise.

● *"Exercise is a great way to meet people."*

Many activities provide opportunities to meet people, make friends, and strengthen friendships. Aerobic dance and team sports are two examples of social activities.

● *"I think exercise is really fun."*

You might think that many kinds of physical activity are simply fun. Many people feel they would exercise even if it did not improve their health. Participating in an activity you enjoy also helps reduce stress.

● *"I enjoy the challenge."*

Sir Edmund Hillary was asked why he climbed Mt. Everest. "Because it was there," was his reply. Climbing Mt. Everest was a challenge. The challenges of various activities help make exercise enjoyable.

● *"I make exercise part of my day."*

Some people enjoy a regular exercise routine. Winning a game or a race is less important to them than the enjoyment of a daily workout.

● *"I like the competition sports and activities provide."*

Many sports, such as tennis and softball, provide people with a socially acceptable way to compete. These and other sports provide ways for people to test themselves against others, if they enjoy competition. You can even compete against yourself by trying to improve your score or time in an activity.

● *"Exercise is my way of relaxing."*

Exercise is an effective means of relaxation. After doing school work, physical activity can be a good way to "get away from it all." Just as you might read a book to relax after working hard, exercise can help you relax after a mentally draining day.

● *"I think exercise improves my appearance and health."*

Exercising to improve your appearance is one of the most common reasons for exercising. However, while exercise can help you look your best, it cannot completely change your appearance. While exercising to improve your health is a good reason, you should start exercising *before*, not after, you have a health problem.

YOUR OWN ATTITUDES Your attitudes play an important role in exercise. You can determine your attitudes toward physical activity by completing the "How I Feel" questionnaire on worksheet 1-3. It is not important that you have a high score on all questionnaire items. Use the questionnaire to help you evaluate your attitudes and to determine how they might affect your future physical fitness.

WORKSHEET 1-3

Complete the "How I Feel" questionnaire on worksheet 1-3.

CHAPTER REVIEW

MULTIPLE CHOICE

Choose the letter of the best answer.

1. Total fitness (a) is the same as physical fitness. (b) refers to skills only. (c) can be achieved only by the young. (d) includes physical, mental, social, and emotional fitness.

2. Regular physical exercise can help (a) change your heredity. (b) control your heredity. (c) change some characteristics regardless of heredity. (d) change all your characteristics.

3. Cardiovascular fitness is one part of (a) skill-related fitness. (b) health-related fitness. (c) emotional fitness. (d) social fitness.

4. Body fatness is the (a) amount of the body that is fat. (b) percentage of body weight that is fat. (c) total body weight. (d) percentage of body weight that is bone and muscle.

5. The ability to use your joints fully is (a) strength. (b) flexibility. (c) power. (d) speed.

6. The ability to change body position quickly and accurately is (a) agility. (b) power. (c) balance. (d) strength.

7. A strong heart and healthy lungs are necessary for (a) cardiovascular fitness. (b) agility. (c) coordination. (d) speed.

8. A hypokinetic condition is a health problem (a) of the elderly. (b) of infants. (c) related to age. (d) caused partly by lack of exercise.

9. The amount of force your muscles can produce is a measure of your (a) strength. (b) power. (c) muscular endurance. (d) agility.

10. How many parts make up physical fitness? (a) 3 (b) 6 (c) 11 (d) 5

MATCHING

Match the definition in Column I with the term it defines in Column II.

Column I

11. ability to keep an upright posture while standing still or moving
12. ability to use strength quickly
13. ability of your body systems to work together efficiently
14. ability to use your muscles many times without tiring
15. passing of genetic traits
16. amount of time it takes to move once you realize the need to act
17. ability to use your senses together with your body parts
18. amount of force muscles can produce

Column II

a. balance
b. coordination
c. heredity
d. muscular endurance
e. physical fitness
f. power
g. reaction time
h. strength

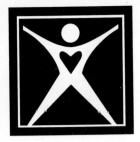

FOCUS ON FITNESS

WARM-UP AND STRETCH

Use these exercises to help you warm up and stretch before vigorous exercise. Keep these guidelines in mind:

● Do the exercises on a soft surface such as carpeting, a mat, a towel, or on grass. Do not do them on a very soft surface, such as a bed.

● Do each stretch at least once and up to three times.

● Stretch slowly and then hold the stretch for a count of 15. Try to stretch the muscles slightly, but do *not* stretch too far. Avoid stretching until you feel pain.

CALF STRETCHER

1. Face a wall and stand 2 or 3 feet away.
2. Reach forward. Touch the wall with your hands.
3. Slowly bend your arms and let your body lean forward. Keep your knees straight and your heels on the floor. *Caution:* Do not arch your back.
4. Turn your toes in slightly. Hold for a count of 15.

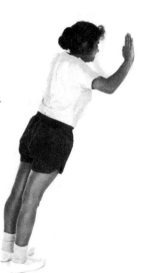

SIDE STRETCHER

1. Stand with your feet about shoulder-width apart.
2. Lean to your left.
3. Reach down with your left hand and over your head with your right arm. Hold for a count of 15.
4. Repeat on your right side. *Caution:* Do not twist or lean your body forward.

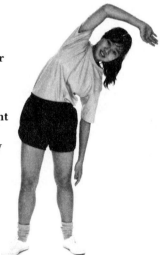

LEG STRETCHER

1. Lie on your back. Lift one leg off the floor with your knee bent.
2. Hug behind the lifted leg with your hands.
3. Slowly straighten your leg as much as you can. You can pull with your arms if you can fully straighten your leg.
4. Try to keep your other leg straight and flat on the floor. Hold for a count of 15.
5. Repeat with your other leg.

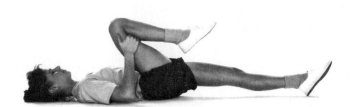

BACK AND HIP STRETCHER

1. Lie on your back. Bend your knees and bring them up to your chest.
2. Reach behind your knees and hug your thighs with your arms.
3. Lift your head and shoulders off the floor as you pull your knees to your chest. Hold for a count of 15.

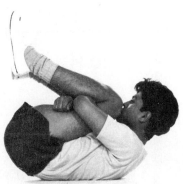

HEART WARM-UP

1. Walk slowly for one minute and then jog slowly for one minute.
2. If you do not have enough room to jog or walk, jog in place for two minutes.
3. Complete the heart warm-up both before *and* after your muscle stretch.

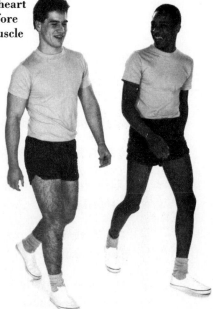

2

EXERCISING SAFELY

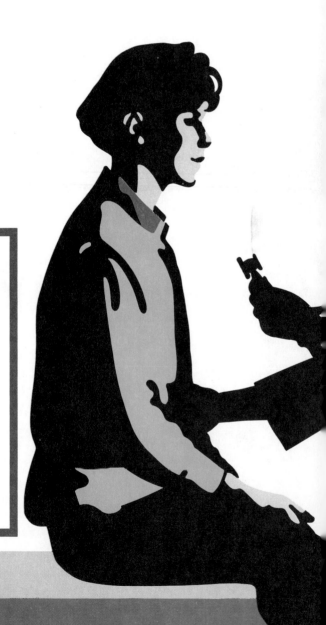

CHAPTER OBJECTIVES

After reading this chapter, you should be able to:

✔ Describe how to prepare yourself for exercise.

✔ List and describe several exercise-related injuries.

✔ Describe how to prevent exercise-related injuries.

✔ Discuss how the environment affects exercise.

Exercise helps improve your health and keep your body systems in good working order. However, exercise is enjoyable and beneficial only when done correctly. Before starting an exercise program, be sure you are prepared to exercise and know how to exercise safely. In this chapter, you will learn about safe exercises. You will also learn about common injuries and how to avoid exercises that can cause injury.

BE MEDICALLY PREPARED

Most schools recommend regular medical examinations for students. Medical examinations help make sure that you are free from disease and can help prevent future health problems. If you have not been physically active for some time, or if you have a known medical condition, consult a doctor before beginning an exercise program. Some schools require a special examination before you participate in a school sports program.

Younger people are less likely to have exercise-related problems than older people. However, even teenagers can have medical conditions that can limit activity. Before starting a vigorous exercise program, a special exercise test is recommended after the age of 45, and for people 35 to 45 with a higher-than-normal risk of heart disease. The test, called an exercise electrocardiogram (EKG), is done on a treadmill and determines the fitness level of the person's heart.

EXERCISE-RELATED INJURIES

If you are beginning a regular exercise program for the first time, you must pace yourself by starting slowly and steadily increasing the length of time and intensity of your exercise. Doing so is very important in avoiding exercise-related injuries that might limit your activity for long periods of time.

COMMON INJURIES By exercising carefully and correctly, you can prevent many injuries. However, injuries still occur in exercise and sports. Sprains, strains, blisters, bruises, cuts, and scrapes are the most common injuries.

A *sprain* is an injury to ligaments and muscles. Ligaments are bands of tissue that connect bones to each other. If a ligament is overstretched, it can cause swelling and pain around a joint. A *strain*, or muscle pull, is an injury to a tendon or muscle. Tendons are bands of tissue that connect muscles to bones. If a muscle or tendon is overstretched, it can cause swelling and pain.

WORKSHEET 2-1

Complete the questionnaire on worksheet 2-1 to assess your readiness for exercise.

More serious, but less common, injuries include joint dislocations and bone fractures. The most common parts of the body injured in exercise and sports are the skin, feet, ankles, knees, and leg muscles. Less likely injuries are to the head, arms, body, and internal organs, such as the liver and kidneys.

Some injuries are called *overuse injuries*. These injuries occur when you do more exercise than your body can handle. Examples include shin splints, "runner's heel," and blisters. These injuries are especially common among long-distance runners and people whose activities cause repeated impact on the feet.

A *side stitch* is a pain in the side of the lower abdomen that a person might experience while exercising. Side stitches are most common among people who are not accustomed to vigorous exercise. A side stitch is not really an injury because it goes away if you stop exercising or if you continue to exercise moderately. Unless the pain is extreme or persistent, a side stitch is not something to worry about. To help relieve a side stitch, press firmly at the point of the pain with your hand while bending forward or backward.

Many of the "harmful" exercises discussed in this chapter cause injuries known as *microtraumas*. You might not think the exercise is harmful because you do not immediately feel pain or soreness. However, the damage eventually appears. Many adults today are now experiencing back problems, neck aches, and stiff, painful joints caused by harmful exercises done when they were younger.

PREVENTING INJURIES Keep in mind these precautions you can take to reduce your risk of injury:

● **Be fit.** By improving your overall fitness, you will be less likely to injure yourself than if you are not fit.

● **Warm up and stretch.** A warm up and stretch is a set of exercises you do before you begin more vigorous exercise.

● **Start slowly.** If you are just beginning vigorous exercise, start slowly. Do not try to do too much too soon.

● **Use moderation.** About 40 percent of regular runners and 50 percent of aerobic dancers experience injuries at some time. Injuries are usually caused by using a body part too much in a period of time.

● **Exercise correctly.** Certain exercises can cause injuries. In addition, you can injure yourself if you perform physical activities incorrectly. Know an activity's proper technique before starting the activity. For example, using the correct jogging technique helps reduce the risk of injury to your back, legs, and feet.

You can get an idea about your own exercise readiness by completing the Exercise Readiness questionnaire. If you answer *yes* to any questions, you might consult with a medical doctor before beginning an exercise program.

EXERCISE AND WEATHER

Weather plays an important role in determining when and how strenuously you exercise. Use these guidelines when exercising outdoors.

HOT WEATHER Be careful when exercising in hot weather. Hot, humid weather causes your body temperature to rise more quickly than it might in cooler weather. Heat-related conditions, such as *heat exhaustion* and *heat stroke*, can occur if your body temperature rises too high. Symptoms of heat exhaustion and heat stroke are shown in the chart. Follow these guidelines to prevent heat-related conditions:

- **Begin gradually.** As your body becomes accustomed to exercising in hot weather, it becomes more resistant to heat-related injuries. Start with short periods of exercise and gradually increase the amount of time you exercise.
- **Drink water.** During hot weather, your body perspires more than normally to cool itself. Drink plenty of water to replace the water your body loses through perspiration.
- **Wear proper clothing.** Wear porous clothing that allows air to pass through it to cool your body. Wear light-colored clothing. Lighter colors reflect the sun's heat, while darker colors absorb heat.
- **Rest frequently.** Exercise creates body heat. Periodically stop and rest in a shady area to help your body lower its temperature.
- **Avoid extreme heat and humidity.** Exercising during hot, dry weather is not as dangerous as exercising during hot, humid weather. If the temperature is above 90°F, use caution when exercising, even if the relative humidity is low (30 percent or less). If the relative humidity is above 30 percent, use caution even if the temperature is lower.

COLD WEATHER Exercising during cold, windy weather can be dangerous. Extreme cold can result in frostbite or hypothermia. Symptoms of *frostbite* and *hypothermia* are shown in the chart. Keep these guidelines in mind when exercising in cold weather:

- **Avoid extreme cold and wind.** Before exercising, determine not only the temperature but also the wind-chill factor, a combination of the wind and temperature. If the wind-chill factor is below 10°F, exercise with great caution or exercise indoors.
- **Dress properly.** Wear several layers of lightweight clothing rather than a heavy jacket or coat. The clothing closest to your body should be made of absorbent material. The outer layers should be nylon or other material that will stop the wind. Avoid nonporous jackets; they do not let your body release heat. Wear a knit hat, ski mask, and mittens, as needed. Mittens keep your hands warmer than gloves.
- **Avoid exercising in wet, cold, or icy weather.** Special problems can occur during wet, cold weather. Your shoes, socks, and pant legs can get wet, increasing the risk of foot injuries and falls.

Exercise and Weather-Related Conditions

Heat Exhaustion:
- approximately normal body temperature
- pale, clammy skin
- profuse perspiration
- tiredness, weakness
- headache, perhaps cramps
- nausea, dizziness (possible vomiting)
- possible fainting

Heat Stroke:
- high body temperature (might be 106°F or higher)
- skin is hot, red, and dry
- pulse is rapid and strong
- victim may be unconscious

Frostbite:
- skin becomes white or grayish-yellow; looks glossy
- pain sometimes felt early, but subsides later (often no pain at all)
- blisters may appear later
- affected area feels intensely cold and numb

Hypothermia:
- shivering
- numbness
- low body temperature
- drowsiness
- marked muscular weakness
- victim acts confused or disoriented, seems apathetic

EXERCISE AND SAFETY

Several factors can influence the effectiveness and safety of exercise. Keep in mind the factors discussed below:

AIR POLLUTION High levels of air pollution affect your breathing ability. Radio and television stations usually issue warnings when air-pollution levels are high. Avoid exercising outdoors during these times.

ALTITUDE People who live in high-altitude locations are able to exercise with little trouble. However, people who live at lower altitudes might have trouble adjusting to higher altitudes. Even if you are physically fit, allow your body to adjust to higher altitudes by first exercising for short periods of time. For example, snow skiers should ski for only part of the first day or two in order to become accustomed to the higher altitude.

PROPER EQUIPMENT Many kinds of physical exercise do not require special equipment. For example, walking and jogging only require proper clothing and good shoes. Other activities, such as ice skating and bicycling, require equipment that is safe and well cared for. Avoid using equipment that is not in good condition. Be sure protective equipment, such as helmets and body padding, fits properly.

PROPER BREATHING Proper breathing while exercising is important. Sometimes people unintentionally hold their breath while exercising. At other times, they might *hyperventilate*, or breathe too quickly. Breathe at an even, regular rate when exercising; do not hold your breath. In some cases, such as weight training, special breathing techniques are helpful.

HARMFUL EXERCISES

Some popular exercises can be harmful because they can cause muscle strain or joint damage. You might not be aware that an exercise is hurting you because you do not always feel pain immediately. Sometimes the damage is gradual and does not appear until you are older.

For some athletes, it might be impossible to avoid potentially harmful exercises. For example, gymnasts must perform stunts that require back arching; softball and baseball catchers must do full squats. It is especially important that these people do extra flexibility and strength exercises to prepare their bodies for these activities. They should carefully warm up and cool down before and after exercise. If pain occurs when exercising, medical attention should be obtained immediately.

Many safer exercises, based on sound biomechanical principles, can fill the same purpose without injuring you. Avoid the harmful exercises shown on page 17; substitute the safer exercises shown on page 18.

HAVE YOU HEARD?

Biomechanical principles are rules for helping a living machine function efficiently. *Bio* on the front of a word means "life." *Mechanical* means "working like a machine."

WORKSHEET 2-2

Use worksheet 2-2 to assess your exercise environment.

DOUBLE-LEG LIFT AND STRAIGHT-LEG SIT-UP

● Do not lie on your back and lift and lower both legs while they are straight. Do not lie on your back with both legs straight and try to sit up. Your lower back might arch and damage your spinal discs or cause swayback. These exercises can also overstretch your abdominal muscles.

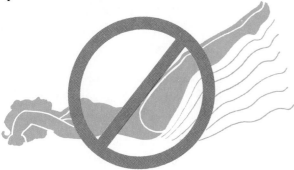

BACK-ARCHING, TRUNK OR NECK CIRCLE, AND ARM CIRCLE (PALMS-DOWN)

● Several exercises make the lower back arch. Most people should avoid these exercises because they tend to stretch the abdominal muscles and can injure the spinal discs. In addition, these exercises might shorten the back muscles, which are already too short in many people. People with swayback, weak abdominal muscles, protruding abdomen, or any back problem should be particularly cautious. Other exercises, such as trunk or neck circling, can injure your spine. Arm circles, with palms turned down, can be harmful to the shoulder joints.

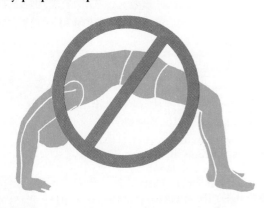

BICYCLE STAND, YOGA PLOUGH, AND HANDS-BEHIND-HEAD SIT-UP

● These exercises make your neck and upper back hyperflex, or bend your head toward your chest more than is safe. Bending your neck too much in these ways can harm the discs and nerves in your upper spine. Ligaments and muscles can also be overstretched, causing humpback and other posture problems.

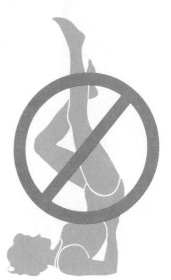

DEEP-KNEE BEND, DUCKWALK, HURDLE SIT, AND TOE TOUCH WITH BOTH LEGS STRAIGHT

● These exercises can cause your knee ligaments to be overstretched. These exercises might also damage your knee joints. Finally, these exercises are even worse when your feet and knees are not aligned. When exercising, do not squat so low that your knees are bent at more than a 90° angle.

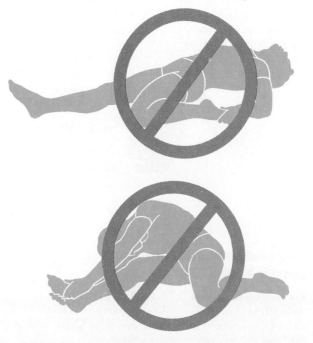

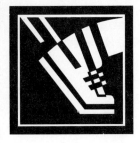

ACTIVITY

SAFE EXERCISES

WORKSHEET 2-3
Use worksheet 2-3 to record your results of this activity.

Exercises such as the ones described here are safe to perform, providing you follow directions. Try each exercise, but remember not to move a body part past the position described in the directions.

TRUNK CURL

● This exercise is sometimes referred to as a "crunch." It strengthens your upper abdominal muscles. Begin by holding your hands and arms straight in front of you. As you improve, you might hold your arms across your chest. When you become very good, you might place your hands on your cheeks. *Caution:* Your feet should not be held while doing a curl.
1. Lie on your back with knees bent and feet close to your buttocks. Place your hands on opposite shoulders.
2. Curl your head and shoulders up only until your shoulder blades leave the floor.
3. Slowly roll back to starting position.

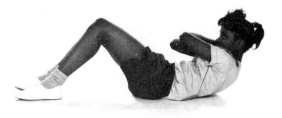

LOWER BODY LIFT

● This exercise helps strengthen your back and hip muscles. You can also do an upper body lift, but be sure to have a partner help you. See page 55 for directions.

REVERSE CURL

● This exercise develops your lower abdominal muscles. A reverse curl can be made more difficult for the advanced exerciser by doing it on an inclined board with your head elevated. *Caution:* Do not lower your legs to the floor or hold your breath.
1. Lie on your back. Bend your knees, placing your feet flat on the floor. Your arms are at your sides.
2. Lift your knees to your chest, raising your hips off the floor.
3. Return to starting position.

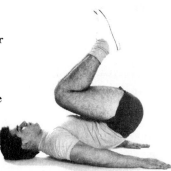

HALF-SQUAT

● Squats are designed to strengthen the muscles on the front of your thighs. Squat halfway down rather than all the way down. Do not bend your knees at more than a 90° angle. Have each knee directly over each foot when squatting.

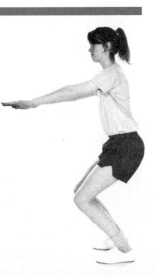

CHAPTER REVIEW

MULTIPLE CHOICE

Choose the letter of the best answer.

1. People who are least likely to need a medical examination before beginning an exercise program are those who (a) have not been physically active for some time. (b) are teenagers. (c) have a medical condition that limits activity. (d) are over 35.

2. The most common injuries that occur in exercise and sports include (a) sprains, dislocations, and head injuries. (b) sprains, strains, and blisters. (c) fractures, dislocations, and strains. (d) fractures, strains, and kidney injuries.

3. A pain in the lower abdomen that occurs while exercising is a (a) side stitch. (b) shin splint. (c) microtrauma. (d) sprain.

4. An injury that is common to long-distance runners is (a) dislocated ankle. (b) broken ankle. (d) side stitch. (d) shin splints.

5. When exercising outdoors in cold weather, wear (a) a heavy coat or jacket. (b) several layers of lightweight clothing. (c) non-absorbent material next to your skin. (d) earmuffs and gloves.

6. Which exercise is safe? (a) trunk curl (b) double-leg lift (c) straight-leg sit-up (d) yoga plough

7. Which exercise is *not* safe? (a) deep-knee bend (b) half-squat (c) trunk curl (d) reverse curl

8. Outdoor exercise is safest in (a) hot, dry weather. (b) hot, humid weather. (c) cool, dry weather. (d) cold, wet weather.

9. When should you do warm-up exercises? (a) before exercising (b) after exercising (c) both before *and* after exercise (d) during exercise

10. A "muscle pull" is another name for a (a) sprain. (b) fracture. (c) strain. (d) microtrauma.

MATCHING

Match the definition in Column I with the term it defines in Column II.

Column I

11. occurs when you do more exercise than your body can handle
12. pain in the side of the lower abdomen
13. injury that does not immediately cause pain or soreness
14. damage to skin and body tissues by exposure to cold
15. condition caused by exposure to cold, characterized by low body temperature
16. breathe too quickly

Column II

a. frostbite
b. hyperventilate
c. hypothermia
d. microtrauma
e. overuse injury
f. side stitch

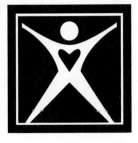

STARTER WORKOUT

This starter workout is designed to help you begin exercising. It can help you prepare for some of the self-evaluations and more advanced exercises in this text. You will probably not find the program difficult if you already exercise regularly. If you do not exercise regularly, you might use this program as your regular exercise program until you can complete the larger number of repetitions shown in this chart. Be sure to warm up before exercising and cool down after exercising.

STARTER WORKOUT

Exercise	Repetitions
Cat Back	3 to 5
Side Leg Raise	5 to 10 (each leg)
Book Curl	5 to 10 (each arm)
Reverse Curl	3 to 8
Knee-to-Nose	5 to 10 (each leg)
Stride Step	3 to 5 (each leg)
Bent Knee Push-Up	3 to 10
Cardiovascular Exercise (choose one)	See directions

SIDE LEG RAISE

1. Lie on your right side. Use your arms to help keep you balanced.
2. Lift your left leg to a 45° angle. Keep your toes and knees pointing forward. *Caution:* Do not rotate your leg so that your knee and toes point toward the ceiling.
3. Lower your leg and raise it again. Roll over and repeat with your right leg.

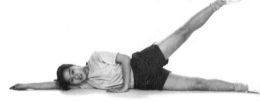

CAT BACK

1. Kneel on the floor and put your hands on the floor in front of you.
2. Lower your head and curve your back upward as high as possible. Then tighten your abdominal muscles and lift as high as you can. Hold for 6 seconds.
3. Lift your head parallel with the floor, lower your back, and relax.

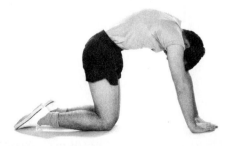

BOOK CURL

1. Stand with your arms straight. Hold a book in each hand, palm up.
2. Lift the books to your chest. Bend each arm at the elbow. Lower your arms and repeat.

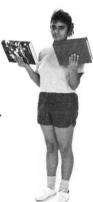

REVERSE CURL

- See page 18 for directions for this exercise.

KNEE-TO-NOSE

1. Kneel on all fours. Lower your head between your arms.
2. Lift one knee to your nose. Then extend that leg behind you until it is straight and parallel to the floor. *Caution:* Do not arch your back or lift your leg higher than parallel to the floor.
3. Repeat several times. Then repeat with your other leg.

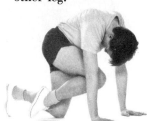

STRIDE STEP

1. Slowly step forward with your left leg. Keep your right leg back. Hold for six seconds.
2. Repeat with your right leg forward and your left leg back. Hold for six seconds.

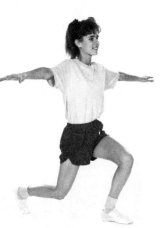

BENT KNEE PUSH-UP

1. Lie face down on the floor with your hands on the floor next to your shoulders. Keep your knees and feet on the floor.
2. Keep your body straight while you push the upper part of your body off the floor.
3. Lower your body until your nose or chest touches the floor.

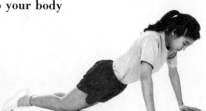

POGO HOP

- This is a cardiovascular exercise.
1. Stand with your knees bent in a half squat. Clasp your hands behind your neck.
2. Put your right leg forward and your left leg back. Jump straight up and move your left leg forward and your right leg back.
3. Continue jumping and changing leg positions. Each time you land, bend your knees to a half squat. Repeat for one minute. You might also do stride steps for one minute, and then pogo hops for two minutes.

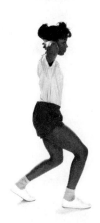

ROPE JUMP

- This is a cardiovascular exercise.
1. Jog while jumping over the rope with one foot and then the other foot. Turn the rope about 120 times per minute. Jump for one minute.
2. Jump on both feet with each rope swing. Jump for two minutes.
3. Alternate the jog step with the two-foot jump for a total of three minutes. Rest by walking for two minutes. Then repeat the jog step and two-foot jump for three minutes.

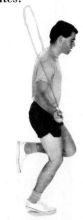

JOG IN PLACE

- This is a cardiovascular exercise.
  At first, jog slowly for twenty paces (each foot touches the floor twenty times). Gradually build up to five minutes. You might also alternate jogging with walking for a total of five minutes. Keep your arms bent and your hands relaxed.

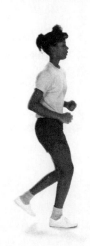

3

PREPARING
FOR EXERCISE

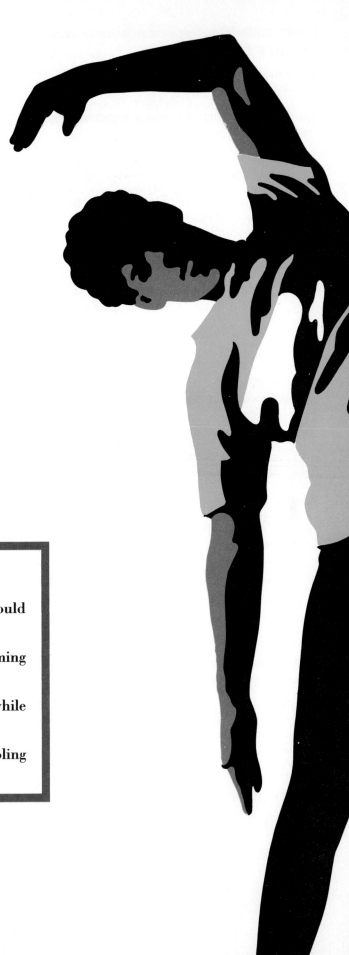

CHAPTER OBJECTIVES

After reading this chapter, you should be able to:

✔ Explain the importance of warming up before exercising.

✔ List guidelines to keep in mind while exercising.

✔ Explain the importance of cooling down after exercising.

A good, safe exercise program includes three stages: a warm-up, a workout, and a cool-down. In this chapter, you will learn about each exercise stage. By preparing properly, all three stages of your exercise program will be more enjoyable. In addition, the benefits of your exercise will increase.

STAGE ONE: WARM-UP

Most experts believe that you should warm up and stretch before starting your *workout*, or the vigorous part of your exercise program. A *warm-up* usually consists of a muscle warm-up and stretch and a heart warm-up. A *muscle warm-up and stretch* includes mild exercises that gently stretch and help contract your muscles.

A warm-up helps reduce your chance of a muscle injury. Your chances of straining a muscle are reduced because the warm-up and stretch increase muscle length. Long muscles are less likely to be strained or "pulled" than short, tight muscles. Warm muscles contract and relax efficiently. In addition, a warm-up and stretch helps make you more flexible. You already know that flexibility is one of the health-related parts of fitness and plays an important part in all kinds of sports and daily activities.

Your heart is also a muscle, and a warm-up helps it get ready for more vigorous exercise. A *heart warm-up* consists of several minutes of walking, slow jogging, or a similar activity that prepares your heart for more vigorous exercise. The importance of heart warm-up increases as you become older. A person with a heart condition, even if it is unknown, is less likely to have discomfort during exercise than a person who has not completed a heart warm-up.

WARM-UP GUIDELINES Use these guidelines to help you properly warm up before exercise:

● Your muscle warm-up should include gentle stretching exercises for each muscle group you will use in your workout. Stretch slowly and easily. Do *not* bounce or jerk or try to stretch too far. The warm-up and stretch on pages 10 and 11 is a good one for most workouts.

● Your muscle warm-up should include a few slow, easy movements that are similar to the activity you will do. For example, if you are going to play baseball, you should warm up your throwing arm. Start by making a few easy, short throws. Gradually work up to longer, harder throws as your arm gets warmer and more limber.

● Your heart warm-up should last between one and three minutes. It might include walking, slow jogging, slow swimming, slow bicycling, or a similar activity. Your goal is to gradually increase your heart rate.

● Some experts think that a heart warm-up should be done both before *and* after a muscle warm-up. They believe that a heart warm-up before a workout increases the blood supply to the muscles, thus raising muscle temperature. Stretching exercises then are more effective because "warm" muscles stretch more easily than "cool" muscles. After the muscle warm-up, a second heart warm-up prepares the heart for vigorous activity.

STAGE TWO: WORKOUT

Your workout is the vigorous part of your exercise program. A workout might be playing a sport, jogging, aerobic dance, or any other physical activity. What you wear can help make exercise more comfortable and enjoyable.

DRESS PROPERLY Consider these guidelines when choosing exercise clothing:

● Wear comfortable clothing. Tight clothing can restrict your blood flow or limit your motion during vigorous exercise. Your body cools itself better if your clothing is not too tight. Expensive exercise clothing is *not* necessary.

● Wear socks. Thick sports socks provide a cushion, help prevent blisters, and absorb perspiration.

● Wash your exercise clothing regularly. Clean clothing is more comfortable and more attractive to other people.

● Dress in layers when exercising outdoors. By dressing in layers, you can remove layers of clothing as you become warmer while exercising.

HAVE YOU HEARD?

The heart of a well-trained athlete beats only half as often as the heart of an average adult. The pulse rate of most adults when they are resting is 70 to 80 beats per minute. Some athletes have pulses as low as 35 to 45 beats per minute.

WEAR PROPER SHOES Most people can use a good pair of "multi-purpose" exercise or sport shoes. However, if you plan to do extensive running or special activities, such as aerobic dance, you might prefer shoes designed for these activities. If you have previously injured your ankles, wear high-top shoes, especially for activities such as basketball and racquetball. Use these guidelines when selecting exercise shoes:

● Try on the shoes before buying them. Wear the socks you normally wear for exercise when trying on shoes. Move around to see how the shoes feel. The shoes should not be too heavy because extra weight makes exercise more tiring.

● Leather or cloth shoes are preferred over vinyl or plastic shoes. Vinyl or plastic shoes do not let air pass through to help cool your feet. Your feet tend to perspire more in vinyl or plastic shoes.

● Shoes do not have to be expensive. However, avoid buying shoes to save a few dollars if they do not have the features of a good exercise shoe. Look for shoes with the features shown here.

STAGE THREE: COOL-DOWN

After working out, your body needs to gradually cool down and stretch to help it recover from vigorous exercise. The *cool-down* has two parts: a heart cool-down, and a muscle cool-down and stretch.

A *heart cool-down* can help keep you from becoming dizzy or even fainting after vigorous exercise. Your heart and blood vessels recover more efficiently if you move rather than sit down or lie down after exercising. Walk, jog slowly, or perform some other slow-moving activity to help your heart and blood vessels return to normal.

Some experts believe that vigorous exercise, especially bouncing stretches, causes small *muscle spasms* or cramps. You can relieve spasms or cramps by stretching slowly. A *muscle cool-down and stretch* slowly stretches the muscles used in your work-out. Your heart cool-down also helps your muscles cool gradually. By doing so, you help reduce muscle soreness and stiffness after exercise. Cooling down now might prevent soreness later. However, a cool-down and stretch cannot prevent all soreness. The best way to prevent muscle soreness is to not overdo exercising.

COOL-DOWN GUIDELINES Use these guidelines when cooling down:
● Do a heart cool-down before stretching your muscles. Start your heart cool-down immediately after stopping vigorous exercise. Your cool-down should last from one to three minutes.
● Your muscle stretch can be the same stretching exercise you did as a warm-up. Stretch slowly without bouncing. Stretch the muscle groups that you used vigorously in your workout.

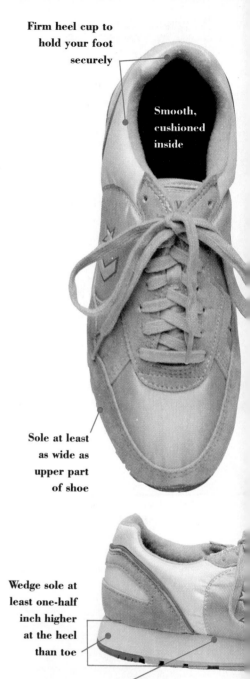

Firm heel cup to hold your foot securely

Smooth, cushioned inside

Sole at least as wide as upper part of shoe

Wedge sole at least one-half inch higher at the heel than toe

Good arch support

ACTIVITY

COUNTING HEART RATE

WORKSHEET 3-1

Use worksheet 3-1 to record your results of this activity.

Before you can determine how a cool-down helps you recover from exercise, you must first learn to count your heart rate.

COUNTING HEART RATE Follow these steps to take your resting pulse:
1. Place your three middle fingers on the side of your throat near your Adam's apple. Press lightly and move your fingers until you locate your pulse.
2. Use a clock or watch to count your pulse for one minute. Try taking your pulse twice. Write your heart rate on your worksheet.
3. Have a partner take your pulse. Try taking your pulse twice. Write your heart rate on your worksheet.

HEART RATE AFTER MILD EXERCISE (no cool-down) You already know that exercise increases your heart rate. When you slow or stop your exercise pace, your heart will also slow. Follow these steps to determine your heart rate after mild exercise:
1. Walk and jog slowly for two minutes.
2. Immediately after walking and jogging, find your neck pulse. Count your pulse for one minute. Write your heart rate on your worksheet.

HEART RATE AFTER VIGOROUS EXERCISE (no cool-down) Follow these steps to determine your heart rate after vigorous exercise:
1. Run 50 to 200 yards. Your instructor will determine the distance. Run as fast as you can.
2. Immediately after running, stand erect without moving. Find your pulse and count it for one minute. Record your heart rate.

HEART RATE AFTER VIGOROUS EXERCISE (with cool-down) If you walk to cool down after vigorous exercise, your heart rate should decrease at a quicker rate than if you simply stopped exercising. Follow these steps to determine your heart rate after cooling down:
1. Run 50 to 200 yards, as you did previously.
2. Immediately after running, locate your neck pulse. Count your pulse for one minute as you walk around. Record your heart rate.
   Compare your heart rates. Which rate is highest? Which is lowest? How does a cool-down help lower your heart rate after exercise?

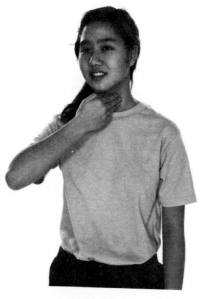

Finding the neck pulse

BASIC EXERCISE SUGGESTIONS

Keep these suggestions in mind when designing your workout. They will help you meet your fitness and exercise goals.

- **Be realistic.** You probably have some very specific goals in mind for your workout. You might want to build muscle, lose body fat, or improve your cardiovascular fitness. Make sure that your goals are realistic. A realistic goal is one that you can really expect to accomplish within three to six weeks. Meeting realistic goals makes you feel successful and good about yourself. Once you reach a realistic short-term goal, you may want to set a long-term goal. Realistic *short-term* goals can help you reach bigger *long-term* goals that might now seem impossible.

- **Evaluate your progress.** In later chapters you will learn how to evaluate your own fitness. Once you have tested each part of fitness, set some realistic goals for each fitness part. By writing down your test results before you start, you can compare them with the results when you test yourself at a later time. The improvement you will see can be very rewarding. However, do not test yourself too often because it takes time to see fitness improvement.

- **Exercise with friends.** Some people are more faithful about exercising regularly if they have someone else to exercise with them. Friends can encourage each other to keep up their exercise. However, remember that friends are there for companionship, *not* to compete. Do not make exercise into a contest to see who can run fastest, lift the most, or do the most repetitions. Each person should exercise at his or her own level.

HAVE YOU HEARD?

A goal is a target to aim for, something to work toward. Short-term goals are ones that can be reached in a short time, such as a few hours, days, or weeks. Long-term goals take more time to reach, maybe months or years. Setting goals can help you stay active and achieve good fitness.

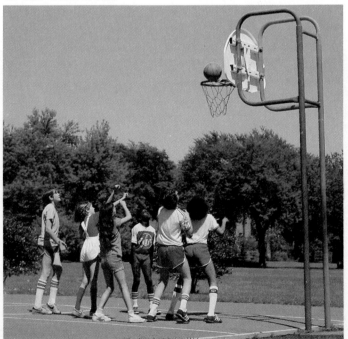

Exercising with friends

● **Have fun.** If you enjoy exercise, you will continue it. Enjoyment is one of the reasons many people participate in sports and other kinds of physical activities.

● **Choose activities you enjoy.** To build total physical fitness you might need to do some exercises you do not particularly enjoy. To stay active throughout your life, your exercise plan should include activities that you enjoy.

● **Plan variety.** Doing the same activity each day can become boring. Try a new or different activity occasionally to keep you interested in exercise. Variety can keep exercise fun and interesting.

● **Select a good time for exercise.** Some people feel that early morning is the best time to exercise. You are fresh early in the morning and exercising can help you feel even more energetic. Other people prefer to exercise at mid-day. Exercising before a light lunch can help you feel more energetic for the rest of the day. Sometimes your efficiency seems to decrease in the afternoon, especially after a large noon meal.

Still other people prefer to exercise before an evening meal. These people say that exercise helps renew their energy after a long day. Finally, some people feel that the best time for exercise is in the evening, after their evening meal has been digested.

Probably more important than when you exercise is that you set aside a regular time as your exercise time. Just as you set aside time to brush your teeth each day, you should set aside an exercise time. The best time of day is what works best for you. If you set an appointment with yourself for exercise, and keep the appointment regularly, you have chosen a good time.

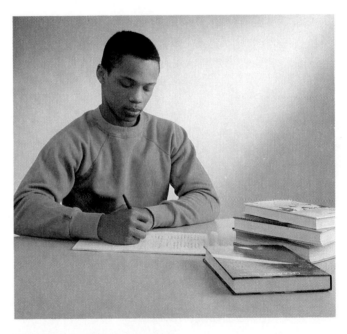

Making a fitness plan

CHAPTER REVIEW

MULTIPLE CHOICE

Choose the letter of the best answer.

1. During vigorous exercise, which muscle condition is *least* likely to result in pulled muscles or muscle strain? (a) cold muscles (b) contracted muscles (c) warm muscles (d) tight muscles

2. How many minutes should a heart cool-down last? (a) 1 to 3 (b) 3 to 5 (c) 4 to 6 (d) 5 to 7

3. What are the benefits of two heart warm-ups, rather than one, before a workout? (a) cool muscles (b) contracted muscles (c) increased blood to muscles (d) increased energy

4. Leather or cloth sports shoes are preferred because they (a) cost less. (b) are easier to fit. (c) keep your feet cooler. (d) look better.

5. What might result from vigorous activity consisting of bouncing stretches? (a) short muscles (b) cold muscles (c) stretched muscles (d) muscle spasms

6. How soon after vigorous exercise should you start your cool-down? (a) immediately (b) as soon as your heart beat returns to its normal rate (c) within 5 minutes (d) within 10 minutes

7. Which is *not* considered one of the stages in a safe exercise program? (a) cool-down (b) timing (c) warm-up (d) workout

8. After vigorous exercise, which best helps your heart and blood vessels return to normal quickly? (a) sit down (b) lie down (c) breathe deeply (d) move about in a slow activity

9. How many weeks does it take a person who is exercising regularly to accomplish some specific fitness goals? (a) 1 (b) 1 to 2 (c) 2 to 3 (d) 3 to 6

10. Which activity is most suitable as a heart warm-up exercise? (a) running (b) walking (c) rapid jogging (d) lifting weights

MATCHING

Match the definition in Column I with the term it defines in Column II.

Column I

11. includes both a muscle warm-up and stretch and a heart warm-up

12. includes both a heart cool-down and muscle cool-down and stretch

13. cramps that might occur after strenuous exercise

14. consists of several minutes of walking, slow jogging, or similar activity

15. prevents dizziness after vigorous exercise

Column II

a. cool-down

b. heart warm-up

c. heart cool-down and stretch

d. muscle spasms

e. warm-up

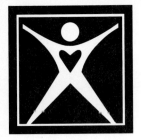

FOCUS ON FITNESS

JOGGING

More than 6 million people in the United States jog for exercise. Many more people could learn to enjoy this excellent cardiovascular exercise if they knew how to jog properly. If you plan to start jogging, use the following biomechanical principles to improve your own jogging technique.

FOOT PLACEMENT The foot action for jogging is not the same as for fast running. In fast running, your weight is mainly on the front of your foot. In jogging, you land on your heel or on the entire foot. Then you rock forward and push off with the ball of the foot, followed by the toes. Jogging improperly can cause injuries, such as sore shins, sore calves, or even a sore back.

LEG MOVEMENT AND STRIDE Swing your legs and feet straight forward. Do not let your feet turn out to the sides. Feet and legs out of alignment cause unnecessary strain on your joints and muscles. When jogging, step farther than your normal walking step.

ARM SWING Swing your arms straight forward and backward; do *not* swing them across your body. Keep your arms bent at the elbows, and hands relaxed. Try to keep your shoulders relaxed.

USING YOUR BODY Keep your trunk fairly erect when jogging. Do not lean forward as you would when starting running fast.

JOGGING GUIDELINES Consider these guidelines for jogging:
• **Learn your own best pace.** Learn how fast or slow you should jog to raise your heart rate to the appropriate level. A correct jogging pace differs for each person. Find your own pace; do not try to jog at someone else's pace, especially if it is faster than your own pace.
• **Avoid running on hard surfaces.** If possible, jog on a running track, grassy places, or dirt paths. These surfaces have more "give" than concrete sidewalks and put less stress on your feet and legs. If you jog indoors, try to jog on a wooden floor rather than on concrete.

JOGGING PRACTICE

Work with a partner to practice the jogging techniques discussed above. Jog about 100 yards twice while your partner stands behind you and checks your technique. On your first jog, your partner should answer these questions to check your feet and legs:

1. Does your heel or whole foot hit the ground first?
2. Do you push off with the ball of the foot?
3. Do your legs and feet swing and land straight ahead?
4. Is your stride longer than walking stride?

During your second jog, your partner should answer these questions to check your arms and body:

1. Are your elbows bent properly (90°) with your hands relaxed?
2. Do your arms swing straight forward and backward?
3. Are your head and chest up?
4. Is your body leaning only slightly?

Discuss your assessment with your partner. Then have your partner jog twice while you evaluate your partner's technique. Practice trying to correct your technique, and then check each other again. Both you and your partner may jog more than twice if necessary.

JOGGING WORKOUTS

Try one or more of these workouts after you have practiced your jogging technique:

BEGINNER'S WORKOUT Run for 15 minutes at your correct heart rate. Use your watch to keep track of how long you run. How long you run is more important than how far. Set your own course. By using time instead of distance, you can jog anywhere. Try to jog half the time away from your starting point and the other half returning to your starting point. If you are not somewhere near your starting point at the end of 15 minutes, walk back to it.

TRAILBLAZING WORKOUT Trailblazing is jogging while trying to follow a trail. It is based on "trailblazing" by pioneers who had to locate signs to stay on the trail. Someone should prepare signs with arrows or other indicators designating the trail. Then try to follow the trail without making an error.

JOG TO THE FRONT Jog with two or three other people of similar ability. Jog in a single-file line. Periodically, the person at the front of the line raises his or her right hand. Then the last person in line jogs quickly to the front of the line. Repeat this procedure several times. This activity gives each person an opportunity to jog both slowly and more quickly.

4

HOW MUCH EXERCISE IS ENOUGH?

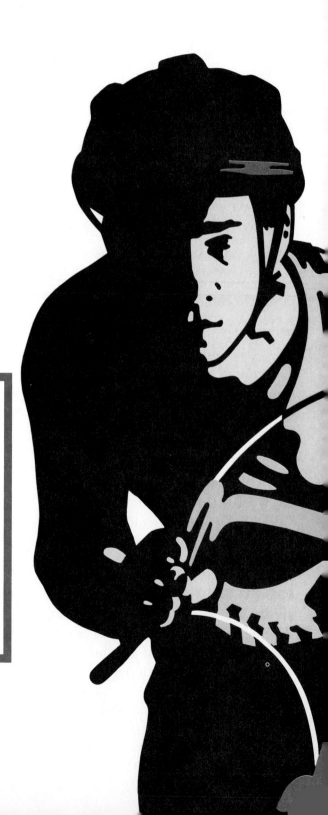

CHAPTER OBJECTIVES

After reading this chapter, you should be able to:

✔ Name and discuss the three basic exercise principles.

✔ Explain the FIT Formula.

✔ Discuss how much exercise is enough for you.

✔ Determine how physically fit you should be.

You must exercise correctly in order to benefit from exercise. A sound exercise program is built on three basic principles: overload, progression, and specificity. In this chapter, you will learn about each exercise principle and how much exercise is enough for your needs.

PRINCIPLE OF OVERLOAD

The only way you can improve your fitness through training is to do more exercise than you normally do. The *principle of overload* involves an increase in exercising, or exercising more than you normally do. By exercising more, or overloading, you build fitness. If you do not exercise more than normal on a regular basis, your fitness decreases.

PRINCIPLE OF PROGRESSION

The *principle of progression* is increasing exercise gradually. After a while, your body will adapt to your exercise (load) so that your exercise is too easy. When this happens, increase your exercise slightly until you adapt to the new load.

The minimum amount of overload necessary to build physical fitness is called the *threshold of training*. Exercising above the threshold of training builds fitness. However, it is possible to exercise too much—or go above your "target ceiling." If you overload too much, your muscles might become sore or you might injure yourself.

Ideally, you should exercise in your *target fitness zone*—above your threshold of training and below your target ceiling. When you exercise in your fitness target zone, you are doing the right amount of exercise to build fitness; you are following the principles of overload and progression.

THE FIT FORMULA

The principle of overload states that you must exercise more than normal to build fitness. The principle of progression states that you should gradually increase your exercise in order to stay within your fitness target zone. You can use the *FIT Formula* to help you determine how much exercise is enough for you to build good fitness.

FREQUENCY *Frequency* refers to how often a person exercises. You must exercise often enough to build fitness. For exercise to be of benefit, you need to exercise at least three times a week. Not exercising often enough can cause problems. For example, a person exercising only one day a week will not improve in fitness and will probably be very sore and stiff after that one day of activity.

INTENSITY *Intensity* refers to how hard a person exercises. Exercising too easily or not enough will not improve your fitness. In fact, your fitness might even decrease. On the other hand, extremely vigorous exercise can be harmful, especially if you have not exercised regularly or if you are not in good health. In addition, too much exercise can make you sore and increase your risk of injury.

TIME *Time* refers to how long a person exercises. You must exercise in your target zone at least 15 to 30 minutes at one time to improve your fitness. Most parts of fitness are not improved by exercising for only a few minutes several times per day. Exercise benefits come from a gradual increase in the time spent exercising.

PRINCIPLE OF SPECIFICITY

The *principle of specificity* states that you must do specific activities to build specific parts of fitness. For example, an exercise to improve strength may not improve flexibility or agility. A specific type and amount of exercise is needed to develop each of the eleven parts of fitness; each exercise puts different demands on your body.

You can see from the principle of specificity that the FIT Formula must be applied differently to each part of physical fitness and for each body part. The chart on page 35 shows how the FIT Formula is applied to each of the five parts of health-related fitness. You will learn more about the threshold of training and target zones in Chapters 6 through 10.

F I T

Part of Fitness	Frequency (how often)	Intensity (how hard)	Time (how long)
Cardiovascular Fitness	**Threshold:** three days per week **Target:** five to six days per week	Make the heart beat faster than normal—for teenagers, about 135-165 beats per minute.	**Threshold:** 15 minutes **Target:** 30 minutes or more
Muscular Strength	**Threshold:** three days perweek **Target:** every other day	Lift more weight than you normally lift. Increase the amount of weight you lift each time, but build up slowly.	**Threshold:** Repeat each exercise three to eight times. **Target:** Do three sets of three repetitions for each exercise.
Muscular Endurance	**Threshold:** three days per week **Target:** five or six days per week	Continue an exercise longer than usual. Increase the number of times you repeat an exercise, but build up slowly.	**Threshold:** Repeat exercises using only certain body parts for one minute—repeat exercises using the whole body eight times. **Target:** Several minutes for exercises using only certain body parts—up to 25 times for exercises using the whole body.
Flexibility	**Threshold:** three days per week **Target:** daily	Stretch muscles longer than usual, but do so slowly.	**Threshold:** Stretch and hold an exercise for 10 to 15 seconds. **Target:** Repeat three different times, resting muscles between stretching.
Body Fatness	**Threshold:** three days per week **Target:** daily	Exercise enough to burn extra Calories and lose extra body fat. Exercise enough to stay lean.	**Threshold:** 15 to 30 minutes **Target:** more than 30 minutes

HAVE YOU HEARD?

To improve fitness test scores, the fit formula should be followed. Scientists have found that less vigorous exercise can provide important health benefits. For example, walking 30 minutes each day can reduce the risk of heart disease.

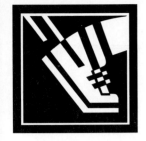

ACTIVITY

TARGET HEART RATE

WORKSHEET 4-1

Use worksheet 4-1 to record your resting heart rate and to calculate your target heart rate.

Each part of physical fitness has target rates. Frequency and time are relatively easy to determine. Intensity is more difficult to determine. Use this activity to familiarize yourself with the concept of target heart rate—a way to determine cardiovascular fitness. *Note:* Before doing this activity, exercise several days a week for several weeks.

COUNTING YOUR PULSE Count your pulse to find how high your heart rate rises during an activity. Follow these steps:

1. Start counting immediately after the activity.

2. Practice finding your pulse within 5 seconds or less. Count your pulse for 15 seconds. Multiply that number by 4 to find your heart rate per minute. This number is your intensity level for that activity.

DETERMINING TARGET HEART RATE Your resting heart rate is the number of times your heart beats per minute when you are still. Follow these steps to determine how high to raise your heart rate while jogging so that you are exercising within your fitness target zone:

1. Find your resting heart rate on the chart. Then find your aerobic intensity level. If you have not exercised at least 3 days a week for the last month, use the "Beginner" column. If you have been active, use the "Regular" column. *Note:* People over age 20 should reduce their intensity by 5 beats for every 10 years over age 20. Record your level on your worksheet.

2. Jog 200 to 500 yards, as set by your instructor. Jog at a steady pace the entire distance. Be especially careful not to run faster at the end of the jog. You want your heart rate after exercise to be as near as possible to your heart rate during exercise. Jog slower than you think you should the first time you jog. Do not race. This activity is to help you find your own best intensity level.

3. Immediately after jogging, count your 15-second heart rate. Multiply by 4 to get your heart rate in beats per minute.

4. Try jogging that distance 3 times. Rest several minutes between jogs. After each jog, record your heart rate on your worksheet. On the second and third jog, try to jog at a pace that will raise your heart rate as near as you can to your own target heart rate.

Target Heart Rates

(beats per minute)		
Resting Heart Rate	Beginner	Regular
Below 50	135–140	145–150
51–70	140–145	150–155
71 and over	145–150	155–160

HOW MUCH FITNESS IS ENOUGH?

Most experts agree that you should have enough physical fitness to:
- reduce your risk of health problems.
- be able to enjoy your free time.
- meet emergencies.
- look your best.
- work effectively.

During this course, you will learn self-evaluations that you can use to determine your physical fitness. A self-evaluation is a test you give yourself to learn more about your physical fitness. You will use rating charts to determine whether or not your fitness is as good as it should be, and whether you are fit enough to meet the goals listed above. You can use worksheet 4-2 to estimate your fitness levels at this time. Keep the worksheet for future comparisons.

LOW FITNESS Experts believe that people who have low ratings for health-related fitness have an above-average risk of certain health problems. People in the low fitness category might not look their best, feel their best, nor work and play most efficiently.

MARGINAL FITNESS People who have marginal ratings are more fit than people with low fitness ratings. Moving from the low to the marginal rating shows important progress in fitness. However, people with marginal ratings must continue to work to progress to the good fitness category.

GOOD FITNESS A good fitness rating indicates that you probably have the necessary amount of fitness needed to live a full, healthy life. In fact, achieving good fitness is the goal of most people. If you want to be a good performer at a certain activity or sport, you will want to further develop your fitness.

HIGH PERFORMANCE Most experts agree that a high performance rating is *not* necessary for good health, meeting normal daily emergencies, and daily activities. However, some people work to achieve a high performance fitness rating. Suppose you want to be an athlete, such as a skilled performer in a sport, or a fast runner, or you want to perform some exceptional physical task. Achieving a high performance fitness rating can increase your chances of success.

SUPER FITNESS People sometimes make the mistake of trying to achieve a "super rating." They think that if some fitness is good, more fitness must be even better. However, sometimes super ratings can be harmful. The health problems associated with doing too much exercise are discussed in later chapters.

WORKSHEET 4-2

Use worksheet 4-2 to estimate your fitness levels.

HAVE YOU HEARD?

Because people have learned about the importance of fitness, the number of people who use part of their free time to do regular exercise has almost tripled in the last twenty years.

PERSONAL FITNESS GOALS

For most people, a reasonable goal is to achieve good fitness in all five parts of health-related fitness. If you have a special interest in athletics, or hope to have a physically demanding occupation, you might work to achieve a high performance rating.

While regular exercise can improve the fitness of anyone, some people find it easier to become fit than others. Heredity plays an important role in determining your fitness, especially for skill-related physical fitness, such as reaction time and how fast you can run. Heredity refers to the characteristics with which you are born. Certain physical characteristics are inherited. For example, some people are taller than others because their parents were tall. Similarly, some people have more muscle fibers, bigger bones, fewer fat cells, or faster reaction times than other people do. Consider these points as you try to determine your goals:

- Try to achieve good fitness ratings for each part of health-related fitness. You might not achieve this goal immediately, but with regular exercise you can do it.
- Avoid comparing yourself to other people. Remember that heredity plays a major role in body shape and physical fitness. What really counts is how you compare to yourself. Use the self-evaluations in this book to periodically measure your fitness. Gradually, with regular exercise, you will see improvement.
- If you want to achieve a high fitness level, use your self-evaluations to decide which sports or activities are best for you. For example, while you might not have inherited the ability to run fast, you might have very good strength, coordination, or some other ability.
- Measure yourself on as many different traits as possible. The more information you have about your fitness, the more accurate your overall fitness assessment will be.

Sometimes another person scores as well as you do on a fitness test even though the person does *not* exercise regularly. Such results might cause the other person to assume that he or she does not need to exercise regularly. In addition, such results might discourage you. You might think, "It's not fair. I exercise hard and that person doesn't, and I still am not as fit as that person." Do not allow yourself to be discouraged by someone else's results. Remember that your fitness will continue to improve if you exercise regularly.

Both fitness *and* exercise are important. Good fitness ratings will help you achieve the health benefits discussed earlier. However, regular exercise is also necessary to achieve these benefits. People who perform well due to inherited abilities alone will not benefit as much as people who achieve good fitness by exercising regularly. Over your lifetime, regular exercise and good fitness will pay off for you.

HAVE YOU HEARD?

There are two types of personal fitness goals—physical fitness goals and exercise goals. Exercise goals make good short-term goals. Fitness goals make good long-term goals. Achieving the short-term goal of doing exercise 30 minutes a day, three days a week, can help you meet important long-term physical fitness goals, such as improving your cardiovascular or flexibility test scores.

CHAPTER REVIEW

MULTIPLE CHOICE

Choose the letter of the best answer.

1. Gradually increasing exercise intensity describes the principle of (a) progression. (b) overload. (c) specificity. (d) fitness target zone.
2. Which is *not* one of the principles on which a sound exercise program is built? (a) overload (b) progression (c) specificity (d) fitness target zone
3. Which is *not* one of three items associated with the FIT Formula? (a) time (b) target ceiling (c) frequency (d) intensity
4. How many minutes at a time should you exercise in order to improve your fitness? (a) 3 to 5 (b) 5 to 10 (c) 10 to 15 (d) 15 to 30
5. Which is *not* a desirable rating for health-related fitness? (a) good fitness (b) super fitness (c) fair fitness (d) high performance
6. Which of the following applies to the principle of specificity? (a) type of clothing you wear (b) your strength (c) how hard you exercise (d) type and amount of exercise you do
7. Which might occur if you go above your target ceiling while exercising? (a) sore muscles or injury (b) reduced coordination (c) increased strength (d) nothing
8. Which is most useful for building fitness? (a) comparing your skills to those of someone else (b) fitness self-evaluations (c) good sports equipment (d) specific clothing
9. According to the FIT formula, how often should you do health-related fitness exercises? (a) at least 3 times each day (b) at least 3 days per week (c) daily (d) It varies.
10. How many times a week must you exercise in order for exercise to benefit you? (a) 2 (b) 3 (c) 4 (d) 5

MATCHING

Match the definition in Column I with the term it defines in Column II.

Column I

11. minimum amount of overload needed to build fitness
12. how often a person exercises
13. exercising more than you normally do
14. increasing exercise gradually
15. range from threshold of training to target ceiling

Column II

a. fitness target zone
b. frequency
c. principle of overload
d. principle of progression
e. threshold of training

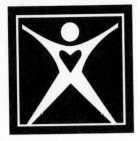

FOCUS ON FITNESS

CIRCUIT TRAINING WORKOUT

Circuit training consists of several different exercises done consecutively. You move from one exercise station to the next. At each station, you complete a certain exercise. When you have completed the exercises at each station, you have completed the exercise "circuit."

You can use circuit training to increase your exercise overload. As you improve at a certain exercise, you can increase the number of times you complete an exercise. You can also try to complete each exercise more quickly. If you try to complete the circuit more quickly, take extra care to do each exercise properly.

Circuit-training exercises should include all parts of fitness and all different body parts. Jump ropes, chin-up bars, and other equipment can be used at the exercise stations. You can perform calisthenics at each exercise station if no special equipment is available. Circuit training is usually planned by an exercise specialist, but you can plan your own circuit training course. Try the sample circuit-training program described here. Remember to warm up before exercising and cool down after exercising.

CIRCUIT TRAINING WORKOUT

Exercise	Repetitions
Body Bender	15 within 2 minutes
Jump Rope	
(jog step)	60 jumps per minute for 2 minutes
(two-foot hop)	60 jumps per minute for 2 minutes
Trunk Curl	5 to 10 within 2 minutes
Bench Step	50 within 2 minutes
Inch Worm	5 to 15 within 2 minutes
Sprint the Lines	6 within 2 minutes
Knee Lift	5 per leg within 2 minutes
Jog in Place	120 steps per minute for 2 minutes

BODY BENDER

1. Stand with feet shoulder width apart.
2. Clasp your hands behind your neck.
3. Bend your trunk sideways to the left as far as possible.
4. Repeat to the right.

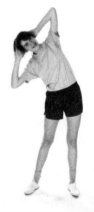

JUMP ROPE

● See pages 146 and 147 for directions for the jog step and the two-foot hop.

TRUNK CURL

1. Lie on your back with your hands folded across your chest.
2. Bend your knees at a 90° angle.
3. Roll your head and shoulders forward and upward. Roll far enough to feel tension in your abdominal muscles. *Caution:* Do not lift your back off the floor.
4. Return to the starting position.

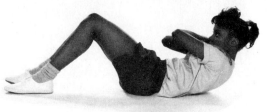

SPRINT THE LINES

1. Run from one line to another 10 yards away.
2. Walk back and repeat.

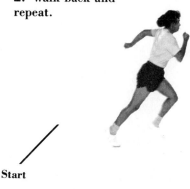

Start

10 yards

BENCH STEP

1. Step up with your right foot, then up with your left foot.
2. Step down with your right foot and down with your left foot.
3. Repeat this 4-count (up, up, down, down) stepping about 24 times per minute.

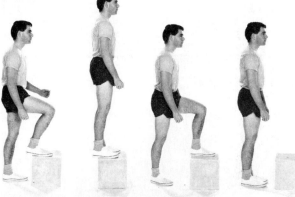

KNEE LIFT

1. Stand with your feet together and arms at your sides.
2. Raise your left knee as high as possible, grasping your thigh with your hands.
3. Pull your knee against your body while keeping your back straight.
4. Return to starting position and repeat with your right knee.

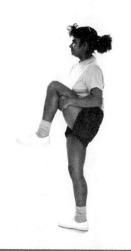

JOG IN PLACE

- Jog in place at a rate of 120 steps per minute.

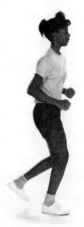

INCH WORM

1. Support your body with your arms and feet in a pushup position.
2. Slowly bring your feet forward as if walking toward your hands, but do not move your hands. Walk forward as far as you can.
3. Slowly bring your feet back to starting position.

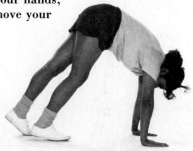

5

EXERCISE AND GOOD HEALTH

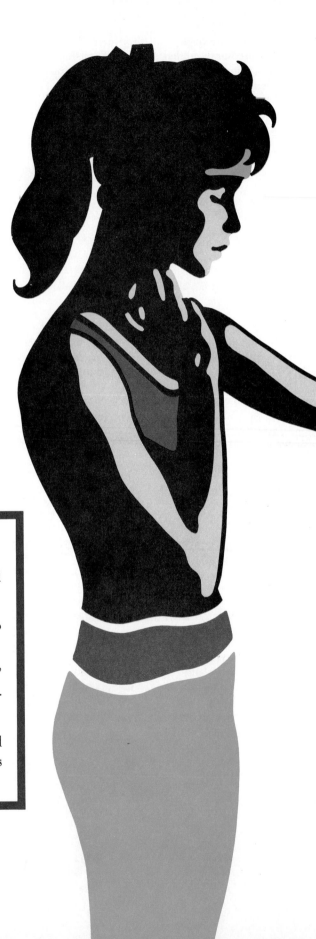

CHAPTER OBJECTIVES

After reading this chapter, you should be able to:

✔ Explain how exercise is related to good health.

✔ Define "hyperkinetic condition" and give two examples of health problems caused by this condition.

✔ Define "hypokinetic condition" and give three examples of health problems caused by this condition.

You already know that regular exercise helps reduce health-related risk factors. In this chapter, you will learn more about the relationship between exercise and good health.

WHAT EXERCISE CAN DO

While exercise will not keep you from getting all diseases, nor prevent or cure infections, it does seems to help some medical problems. Many doctors agree that people with a "low resistance" are more likely to develop infections. Thus, staying fit and healthy might help increase your resistance to infections. Recent research indicates that people who exercise have less risk of certain types of cancer than people who do not exercise. In addition, exercise under medical supervision can help people with some forms of cancer enjoy life more and feel better. On the other hand, rest is most often recommended for a person with an infection. Avoid vigorous exercise when your body is fighting an infection, such as a cold or flu.

Often, teenagers are not very concerned about their health. They think that health problems only affect older people. However, scientists have found that risk of heart disease starts very early in life. By beginning an exercise program when you are young and continuing it on a regular basis, you can reduce your risk of illness throughout your life. Many older people wish they had known about the value of exercise when they were young. Start an exercise program *now* for good health later. By following the FIT Formula, you can reduce your risk of many health problems, look better, feel better, and enjoy life more.

RISK FACTORS

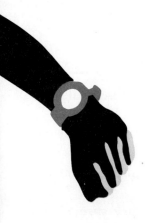

A *risk factor* is anything that increases the chance of somthing occuring. A *controllable risk factor* is something you can act upon to change. Lack of regular exercise is a controllable risk factor. You know that you can reduce your risk by exercising regularly. However, a *noncontrollable risk factor* is one that you cannot change. Age is one example of a noncontrollable risk factor. The activity on page 44 lists examples of both controllable and noncontrollable risk factors.

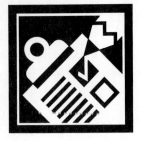

SELF-EVALUATION

DETERMINING RISK OF HEART DISEASE

WORKSHEET 5-1

Complete worksheet 5-1 to help determine your risk factors relating to heart disease.

Read these lists of risk factors. Use them to complete the questionnaire on worksheet 5-1. Find your total score on the rating chart. If you have a high total score for heart disease risk factors, it is important that you change your controllable risk factors. Consult your physician before making decisions about diet and other risk factors.

NONCONTROLLABLE RISK FACTORS
- **Age:** As you get older, your risk of heart disease increases.
- **Sex:** Males have a much greater risk of heart disease than females.
- **Heredity:** People whose parents or grandparents have had heart disease have a higher-than-normal risk.

CONTROLLABLE RISK FACTORS
- **Smoking:** Smokers have twice the risk of heart disease.
- **Fatness:** Overweight people have an increased risk of many illnesses, including heart disease.
- **Diet:** People who eat a high-fat diet have a greater risk of heart or digestive diseases.
- **Stress:** People who have stressful jobs have a higher risk of heart disease.
- **High Blood Pressure:** People with high blood pressure have an increased risk of heart attack and other cardiovascular diseases.
- **Other Diseases:** People with diabetes or ulcers have increased risk of heart disease.
- **Inactivity:** People who do not participate in physical activities and exercise have increased risk of heart disease.

Rating Chart: Risk of Heart Disease

Rating	Noncontrollable Factors Score	Controllable Factors Score	Total Score
High	9 or more	21 or more	31 or more
Above Average	7–8	15–20	26–30
Average	5–6	11–14	16–25
Low	4 or less	10 or less	15 or less

HYPERKINETIC CONDITIONS

Other health problems can arise from excesses or other conditions in a person's lifestyle. Exercising too much or too hard can cause health problems. A *hyperkinetic condition* is a health problem caused by doing too much exercise.

OVERUSE INJURIES An *overuse injury* occurs when you exercise so much that your bones, muscles, and other tissues are damaged. Overuse injuries can also be caused by doing too much exercise without enough rest or doing too much exercise in a short period of time. Overuse injuries include stress fractures, blisters, and shin splints.

ACTIVITY NEUROSIS Neurosis is a condition that occurs when a person is overly concerned or fearful about something. For example, excessive fear of high places is one type of neurosis. People with an *activity neurosis* are overly concerned about getting enough exercise and are upset if they have to miss their regular exercise. In addition, they often continue to exercise even when they are sick or injured.

HYPOKINETIC CONDITIONS

A number of serious health problems are classified as hypokinetic conditions or diseases. A *hypokinetic condition* is one associated with, or caused by, a lack of physical activity or regular exercise. In many cases, cardiovascular diseases and lower-back problems are related to hypokinetic conditions. Physically fit people are less likely to develop hypokinetic conditions.

OBESITY *Obesity* is a condition in which a person has a high percentage of body fat. Often, obesity is the result of a hypokinetic condition. You have learned that having too much body fat increases the risk of heart disease. Being "overfat" increases your risk of other diseases as well. Regular exercise and good eating habits can help reduce excess body fat.

OSTEOPOROSIS *Osteoporosis* is a condition in which the bones become porous and start to lose their strength. Osteoporosis is more common among older people, especially women. The type of bones you will have as an adult are determined by what you do *now.* Regular exercise and a healthful diet (including ample calcium) are the best ways to lower your risk of getting osteoporosis in the future.

INSOMNIA People with *insomnia* have difficulty getting to sleep and staying asleep. This lack of sleep can contribute to physical, mental, and emotional problems. While experts have not proven that exercise can prevent insomnia, studies show that most people believe that they sleep better if they exercise regularly.

CARDIOVASCULAR DISEASES

Cardiovascular diseases are the leading cause of death in the United States. The most common cardiovascular diseases are atherosclerosis, heart attack, high blood pressure, and stroke. In recent years, the number of people with cardiovascular diseases has decreased. This decrease is credited in part to improved medical treatment. People are also more aware of the importance of good nutrition and regular exercise. Still, nearly 5 million Americans suffer from cardiovascular diseases. The American Heart Association reports that as many as 57 million people, including many teen-agers, have high blood pressure.

ATHEROSCLEROSIS *Atherosclerosis* is a disease in which certain substances build up on the inside walls of arteries. This build-up narrows the openings through the arteries. As a result, the heart must work harder to pump blood through these narrowed arteries. Notice in these pictures how an artery can become so narrow that blood cannot flow properly to the heart, brain, and other organs. Atherosclerosis also increases the risk of high blood pressure and blood clots.

Several factors increase a person's risk of developing atherosclerosis. These factors include a high-cholesterol and high saturated-fat diet, obesity, smoking, heredity, and lack of regular exercise. People have control over some factors, and therefore can reduce their risks for atherosclerosis by choosing a healthful lifestyle.

HAVE YOU HEARD?

Studies indicated that 77% of the American soldiers killed in the Korean War (average age: 22) showed signs of heart disease, such as deposits that partly or completely block artery walls. On the other hand, Asian soldiers killed at the same time showed no signs of heart disease.

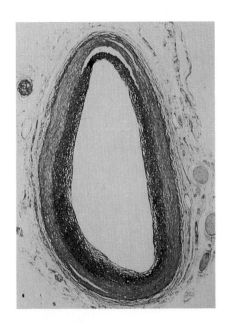

Clear artery

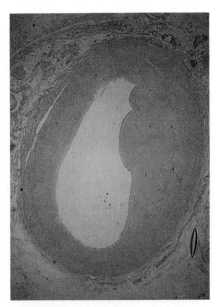

Partially-blocked artery

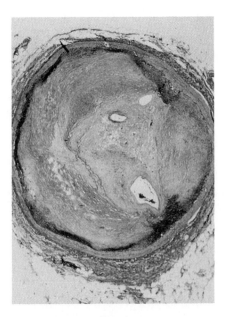

Blocked artery

HEART ATTACK A *heart attack* occurs when the blood supply into or within the heart is severely reduced or cut off. As a result, an area of the heart muscle might die. Coronary arteries can be blocked by atherosclerosis, a blood clot, a spasm in the muscles of the artery, or a combination of these causes. During a heart attack, the heart beats abnormally or even stops beating. Medicines and cardiopulmonary resuscitation (CPR) are often used to stabilize the heartbeat. Doctors prescribe rest, medicines, and a planned exercise program during recovery from a heart attack.

Studies have indicated that people who exercise, or those who are physically active at work, have fewer and less severe heart attacks than people whose work or exercise is less active. However, experts also point out that exercise is only *one* of several factors that can help reduce the risk of heart attack. Other factors include proper diet, no smoking, and weight control. Chapter 6 discusses heart attacks and preventive exercise in more detail.

HIGH BLOOD PRESSURE Each time your heart beats, it forces blood through your arteries. The force with which blood pushes against artery walls is called *blood pressure*. Your *systolic blood pressure* is the highest pressure exerted by the blood within your arteries. Your *diastolic blood pressure* is the lowest pressure exerted by the blood within your arteries. High blood pressure, or *hypertension,* is a disease in which the blood pressure is consistently higher than normal. High blood pressure can weaken arteries and can cause a heart attack, stroke, or kidney damage. The chart shows that the range for normal blood pressure varies. Thus, the range for high blood pressure varies.

Regular exercise is one way to help reduce high blood pressure. Other lifestyle changes might include weight reduction, a low-salt and low-cholesterol diet, no smoking, and stress management. In addition, doctors might prescribe various medicines to lower blood pressure. Finally, regular blood-pressure checks, such as the one pictured here, can help people monitor their blood pressure.

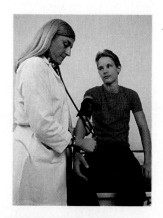

Having blood pressure checked

Blood Pressure Range

	Low Range	"Normal" Range	High Range
Systolic	below 110	between 110–140	140
Diastolic	below 60	between 60–90	above 90

STROKE A *stroke* occurs when oxygen in the blood supply into or within the brain is severely reduced or cut off. A blood clot or atherosclerosis can block any artery that supplies blood to the brain, causing a stroke. A stroke can also occur when an artery in the brain bursts. Some strokes are severe enough to cause death.

Since a stroke damages part of the brain, it also affects a person's ability to move, think, and speak. Physical therapy can help a stroke patient regain the use of some body functions. Unaffected brain areas learn to take over some functions of the damaged brain areas.

Hypertension, atherosclerosis, smoking, and heredity are factors that increase a person's risk of stroke. As pointed out earlier, changes in lifestyle can help reduce the risk of hypertension and atherosclerosis, thereby helping reduce the risk of stroke.

BACK PROBLEMS

Each year, as many as 25 million Americans seek a doctor's care for backache. According to some experts, back pain is the leading medical complaint in the country. Although adults experience most of the back problems, studies show that back problems often begin much earlier in life.

Lordosis, or swayback, is a very common problem among young people. As many as 75 percent of American children fail tests designed to measure muscle weakness that could lead to back problems. Teenagers do almost as poorly in back tests. Examples of muscle groups prone to weakness include the gluteus and abdominal muscles. A weakness of back muscles is not the only cause of back problems. Muscles that are too short can also result in back pain. Examples of these muscles include the iliopsoas, the hamstrings, and back muscles. Bone alignment is affected by the length of these muscles.

Many teenagers who fail these tests are very active people. However, many sports and games do not develop the muscles that can help prevent back problems. Therefore, it is not unusual for basketball players, gymnasts, band members, and other active people to have weak back and abdominal muscles.

Your body parts are balanced like blocks on your legs. Your chest hangs from your spine and is balanced over your pelvis. Your head sits on top of your spine, balanced over the other blocks in the stack. Since your spine is flexible and can move back and forth, the pull of your muscles keeps your body parts balanced. If your muscles on one side are weak and long, while your muscles on the opposite side are strong and short, your body parts are pulled off balance.

Strong, yet not too short, muscles help prevent back problems. You can test yourself in the five areas listed below. People who do poorly on self-evaluations in these five areas have a higher risk of having back problems:

- Strong and long low-back muscles
- Strong gluteus muscles
- Strong and long hamstring muscles
- Long iliopsoas muscles
- Strong abdominal muscles

HAVE YOU HEARD?

The human machine works best when the muscles of the body are balanced both in length and in strength. This biomechanical principle is important to good posture and to the good health of your back.

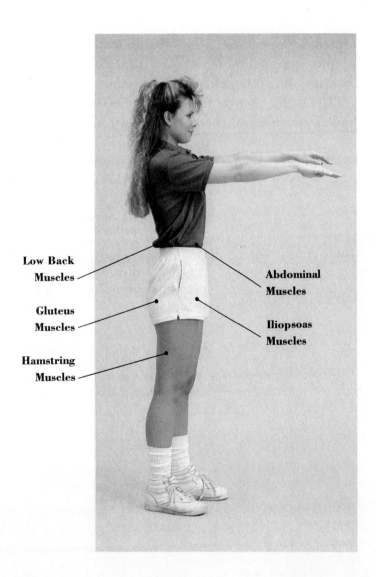

Low Back Muscles

Gluteus Muscles

Hamstring Muscles

Abdominal Muscles

Iliopsoas Muscles

Doing exercises to strengthen these muscles helps prevent back problems.

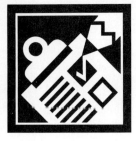

SELF-EVALUATION

THE HEALTHY BACK TEST

WORKSHEET 5-2

Use worksheet 5-2 to record your results of this self-evaluation.

Use this self-evaluation to test the muscles that help support your back. Each part focuses on a certain muscle group. If you do well on this self-evaluation, it is likely that the muscles around your hip joints are functioning well. Follow these directions:

1. Read each set of directions. After a demonstration, try each test.

2. Work with a partner, if possible, when scoring each test.

3. Mark the answer on your worksheet that best describes your performance on each test. Note the points for each answer.

4. Add your points for each of the six tests to get your total score. Then use the rating chart to determine your risk of back problems.

What might you do to reduce your risk of back problems? Do you think your risk will change as you get older?

Rating Chart: Healthy Back Test

Rating	Score
Healthy Back	11–12
Average Risk	8–10
Above Average Risk	6–9
High Risk	below 6

SINGLE LEG LIFT

● This procedure tests your hamstring muscles.
1. Lie on your back on the floor.
2. Lift your right leg off the floor as high as possible without bending either knee.

3. Repeat using your left leg.
4. Score 1 point if you can lift your right leg to a 90° angle to the floor. Score 1 additional point if you can lift your left leg to a 90° angle.

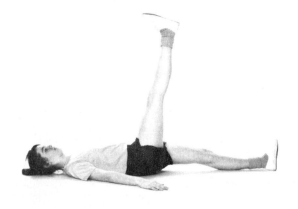

KNEE TO CHEST

● This procedure tests your iliopsoas muscles.
1. Lie on your back on the floor. Make sure your lower back is flat on the floor.
2. Keep your left leg straight and touching the floor. Bring your right knee up until you can hold it tight against your chest. Hold under your knee.

3. Repeat using your left leg.
4. Score 1 point if you can keep your left leg touching the floor while you hold your right leg against your chest. Score 1 additional point if you can keep your right leg touching the floor while holding the left leg against your chest.

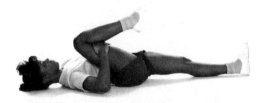

TRUNK LIFT

● This procedure tests your back muscles.
1. Lie face down on the floor.
2. Hold your arms straight out. Lift your upper body off the floor. Hold for 10 seconds.

Caution: Do not lift your hips off the floor.
3. Score 1 point if you can lift your chin 1 foot off the floor. Score 2 points if you can lift your chin 1 foot off the floor for 10 seconds.

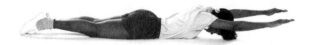

REAR LEG RAISE

● This procedure tests your back muscles.
1. Lie face down on the floor.
2. Lift your straight right leg about 1 foot off the floor behind you. Hold for a count of 10. Then lower your leg.
3. Repeat using your

left leg.
4. Score 1 point if you can lift and hold your right leg 1 foot off the floor and hold for the count. Score 1 more point if you can lift your left leg 1 foot off the floor and hold for the count.

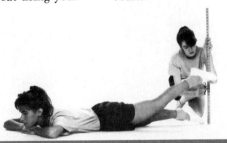

BACK TO WALL

● This procedure tests your back curve.
1. Back up to a wall so that your heels, buttocks, shoulders, and head are against the wall.
2. Try to press your lower back and neck against the wall without bending your knees or lifting your heels off the floor.
3. Have a partner try to place a hand between your back and the wall.
4. Score 1 point if you can press your back against your partner's hand. Score 1 more point if you can press your back against the wall.

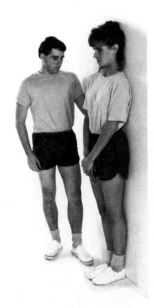

TRUNK CURL

● This procedure tests your abdominal muscles.
1. Lie on your back on the floor with your knees bent.
2. Curl up by rolling your head, shoulders, and upper back off the floor. Roll up only until your shoulder blades

leave the floor.
3. Score 1 point if you can curl up with your arms held straight in front of you *without* having to lift your feet off the floor. Score 2 points if you can curl up with your arms across your chest.

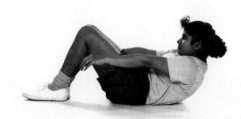

POSTURE PROBLEMS

Strong, long muscles contribute to good posture and help to prevent back problems. Some common posture problems are illustrated here.

Knowing what good posture looks like can help you improve your own posture. Good posture helps you look good, helps prevent back problems, and helps you work more efficiently. Use the self-evaluation on page 53 to check your posture and determine whether or not you have any of the problems shown in the picture.

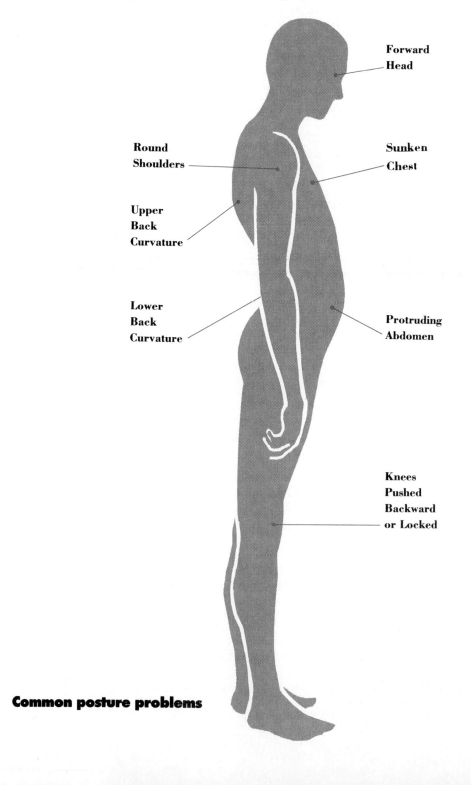

Forward Head

Round Shoulders

Sunken Chest

Upper Back Curvature

Lower Back Curvature

Protruding Abdomen

Knees Pushed Backward or Locked

Common posture problems

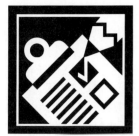

THE GOOD POSTURE TEST

Use this self-evaluation to determine whether your posture is as good as it should be. Practice good posture at all times, not just when taking this self-evaluation. Wear a gym suit, swimsuit, or shorts and a T-shirt when taking this self-evaluation. Work with a partner to determine each other's scores.

1. Stand sideways next to a string hung from at least 1 foot above your head. The string should be weighted at the bottom so that it hangs straight. Position yourself so that the string aligns with your ankle bone.

2. Have your partner answer *yes* or *no* to each question below.

- Head: Is the ear in front of the line?
- Shoulders: Are the shoulders rounded? Are the tips of the shoulders in front of the chest?
- Upper back: Does the upper back stick out in a hump?
- Lower back: Does the lower back have excessive arch?
- Abdomen: Does your abdomen protrude beyond the pelvic bone?
- Knees: Do the knees appear to be locked or bent backwards?

3. Now stand with your back to the string so that the string is aligned with the middle of your back.

- Head: Is more than one-half of the head on one side of the string?
- Shoulders: Is either shoulder higher than the other shoulder?
- Hips: Is either hip higher than the other hip?

4. Total the number of *yes* answers. Check the score against the rating chart. Do you think your posture is as good as it should be? How might you improve your posture all of the time, not just when standing?

WORKSHEET 5-3

Use worksheet 5-3 to record your results for this self-evaluation.

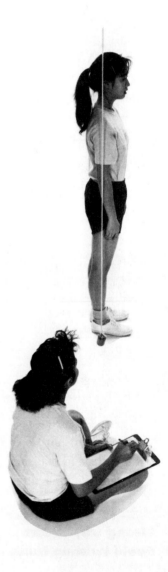

Rating Chart: Good Posture Test

Score (yes answers)	Rating
0–1	Good posture
2–4	Posture can use some improvement
5 or more	Posture definitely needs improvement

BACK CARE AND GOOD POSTURE

If you did not do well on the Healthy Back Test, avoid exercises that require you to arch your back or lift inefficiently with your back muscles. Rather, use the guidelines below and the back exercises in this chapter to help correct or prevent back problems. Since back problems are often related to poor posture, some exercises for improving posture have also been included.

BACK AND POSTURE PRINCIPLES To improve your posture and avoid back strain, keep the following *biomechanical principles* in mind:

● Use the large muscles of the body when lifting. Let the strong leg muscles, not the relatively weak back muscles, do the work.

● When lifting, keep your weight low. Squatting with the back straight and the hips tucked helps keep weight low and makes lifting safer.

● Divide a load to make it easier to carry. For example, carrying two small suitcases, one in each hand, is easier than carrying one larger suitcase with one hand. When carrying your books, carry some in each arm. If you carry your books in one arm, change arms from time to time.

● Avoid twisting while lifting. If you have to turn while lifting, change the position of your feet. It is especially important to avoid twisting your upper body when straightening or bending the spine.

● Push or pull heavy objects rather than lifting them. Heavy lifting can cause injury. Pushing or pulling an object is more efficient than lifting it.

● Avoid a bent over position when sitting, standing, or lifting. The levers of your body, such as your spine, do not work efficiently when you are bent over. When sitting in a chair, sit back in the seat and lean against the back rest. Do not work for long periods of time in a bent over position.

HAVE YOU HEARD?

Many of the same bio-mechanical principles that help avoid poor posture and back problems can aid a person's sports performance and improve his or her work. For example, keeping their weight low helps basketball players play defense. A person sitting in a bent over position while typing will not work as efficiently as when he or she sits properly.

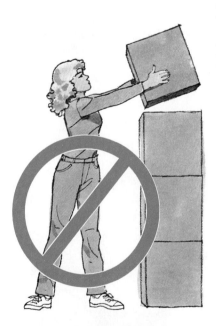

**Wrong way to turn
Avoid twisting trunk**

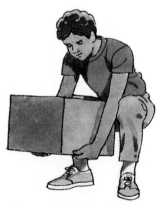

Right way to lift

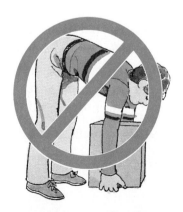

Wrong way to lift

STRENGTHENING EXERCISES FOR GOOD POSTURE AND BACK CARE

Use these exercises to help strengthen the muscles of your back and improve your posture. Remember to move only as far as the directions specify.

TRUNK CURL

- The trunk curl helps strengthen your upper abdominal muscles. See page 51 for directions. Complete up to 10 repetitions.

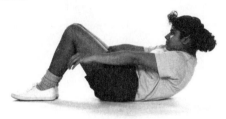

UPPER BODY LIFT

- The upper body lift helps strengthen your back muscles.
1. Lie on a table or bench with a partner holding your legs. Your upper body should hang over the edge.

2. Lift your upper body until it is even with the edge of the table. *Caution:* Do not lift any higher.
3. Lower to beginning position. Repeat up to 10 times.

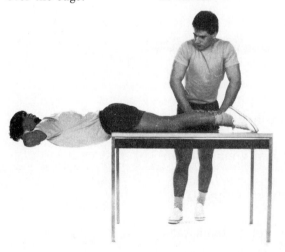

LOWER BODY LIFT

- The lower body lift strengthens your lower back and gluteus muscles.
1. Lie on a table or bench with a partner holding your upper body. If you have no partner, hold under the edge of a table.
2. Lift your hips and legs until your legs are even with the top of the table. *Caution:* Do not lift any higher. You might lift one leg at a time until you are able to lift both legs at one.
3. Lower to beginning position. Complete up to 10 repetitions.

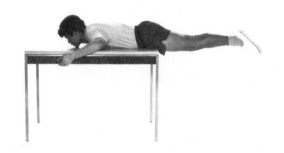

REVERSE CURL

- This exercise helps strengthen your lower abdominal muscles. It is a good exercise to combine with the trunk curl. See page 18 for directions. Complete up to 10 repetitions.

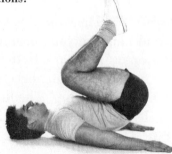

KNEE TO CHEST

● This exercise helps correct or prevent lordosis and backaches.
1. Lie on your back. Bend your right knee to your chest.
2. Grasp the thigh (under the knee) with your arms. Pull it down tight against your chest. Keep your left leg flat on the floor.
3. Return to beginning position. Repeat with your left leg.
4. Pull both thighs to chest and hug them. Repeat exercise up to 10 times.

SINGLE LEG HANG

● This exercise stretches your iliopsoas muscle.
1. Lie on your back on a table or a bench. Your thigh should remain on the table while your knee and the rest of your leg hangs over the edge of the table.
2. Pull your right leg to your chest while keeping your left leg over the edge of the table. Have a partner push your left leg down if it comes up. Hold this position for several seconds.
3. Return to beginning position. Repeat with your left leg. Repeat 10 times with each leg.

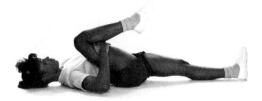

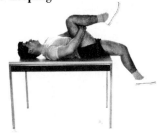

ARM AND LEG LIFT

● This exercise helps prevent rounded shoulders, sunken chest, and rounded upper back.
1. Lie face down with arms stretched in front of you.
2. Raise your right arm, then lower it. Raise your left arm, then lower it. Finally, raise both arms, then lower them.
3. Raise your right leg, then lower it. Raise your left leg, and then lower it.
4. Raise your right arm and right leg, then lower them. Raise your left arm and left leg; then lower them.
5. Raise your left arm and right leg, then lower them. Raise your right arm and left leg, then lower them.
6. Repeat all steps up to 5 times. *Caution:* Do not arch your back.

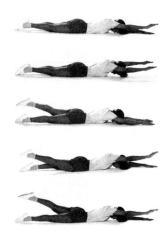

OTHER EXERCISES The exercises listed here can also help strengthen your back and improve your posture:

● **Back Flattener** The back flattener helps strengthen your abdominal muscles. See page 86 for directions.

● **Hip and Thigh Stretcher** The hip and thigh stretcher helps stretch the hip muscles. See page 115 for directions.

● **Trunk Lift** The trunk lift helps strengthen your upper back muscles. See page 79 for directions.

● **Back-Saver Toe Touch** The back-saver toe touch helps stretch your hamstring muscles. See page 115 for directions.

● **Knee-to-Nose Touch** The knee-to-nose touch also helps stretch your lower back. See page 21 for directions.

CHAPTER REVIEW

MULTIPLE CHOICE
Choose the letter of the best answer.

1. Lordosis is (a) curvature of the spine. (b) a type of muscle spasm. (c) protruding abdomen. (d) locked knees.
2. Which back muscle conditions are best for a healthy back? (a) short, strong (b) long, weak (c) weak, short (d) long, strong
3. What should you do in order to turn while carrying a heavy load? (a) First twist your body. (b) Twist your body as you straighten your spine. (c) Use back muscles rather than leg muscles. (d) Change the positions of your fcct.
4. If a person exercises even when ill, he or she might be showing a symptom of (a) a hypokinetic condition. (b) activity neurosis. (c) insomnia. (d) hypertension.
5. Which is *most* likely to be classified among a person's controllable risk factors? (a) amount of stress (b) birth defect (c) age (d) heredity
6. Which is a noncontrollable risk factor? (a) heredity (b) diet (c) amount of exercise (d) amount of stress
7. Avoid vigorous exercise if you are (a) tired. (b) ill. (c) hungry. (d) too busy to exercise.
8. Which muscles are *least* likely to be associated with back and posture problems? (a) bicep (b) abdominal (c) gluteus (d) iliopsoas
9. The force with which blood pushes against the artery walls is known as (a) high blood pressure. (b) blood pressure. (c) systolic blood pressure. (d) diastolic blood pressure.
10. Which indicates a high percentage of body fat? (a) obesity (b) osteoporosis (c) lordosis (d) insomnia

MATCHING
Match the definition in Column I with the term it defines in Column II.

Column I
11. high blood pressure
12. brought on by not enough exercise
13. type of heart disease
14. blisters and muscle pain
15. brought on by too much exercise

Column II
a. atherosclerosis
b. hyperkinetic condition
c. hypertension
d. hypokinetic condition
e. overuse injuries

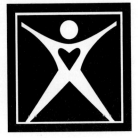

FOCUS ON FITNESS

COOPER'S AEROBICS

Aerobics is an exercise program that was originally developed by Dr. Kenneth Cooper for use by the U.S. Air Force. Now the program is widely used by many other people. Aerobics is well suited for people of all ages and includes many kinds of exercises. Aerobics activities include walking, jogging, running, stationary running, jumping rope, cycling, swimming, racquetball, and basketball.

In this program, you earn points for exercise. Dr. Cooper recommends that men earn at least 35 points per week and women earn at least 27 points per week. You can earn points by doing any of the activities listed here. It has been suggested that you begin by earning 10 to 15 points a week and work up to 27 to 35 points each week. You should earn these points on at least 3 separate days each week.

In a period of 30 to 60 minutes, try to earn 5 points. You may select one or more of the activities on page 59. Remember to warm up before your workout and cool down afterwards.

There are many other activities you can do to earn points. If you are interested in doing Cooper's aerobics as part of your regular exercise program, read *The Aerobics Program for Total Well-Being*, by Dr. Kenneth Cooper.

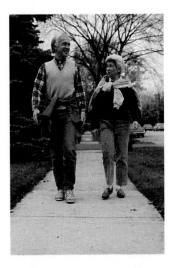

Today, many people do aerobic exercises.

COOPER'S AEROBICS

Points Earned	Walking/Running (1 mile)	Cycling (3 miles)	Swimming (400 yards)
6	less than 6 ½ minutes	less than 9 minutes	less than 6 ½ minutes
5	6 ½–8 minutes	9–12 minutes	6 ½–8 minutes
4	8–10 minutes	12–15 minutes	8–10 ½ minutes
3	10–12 minutes	15–18 minutes	10 ½ minutes
2	12–15 minutes		12–13 ½ minutes
1	15–20 minutes		

Points Earned	Handball/ Basketball/ Racquetball	Stationary Running (steps in 5 minutes)	Rope Jumping (jumps for 5 minutes)
6	35–40 minutes	1,100–1,300 steps	over 600 jumps
5	30–35 minutes	951–1,100 steps	451–600 jumps
4	25–30 minutes	801–950 steps	300–450 jumps
3	20–25 minutes	651–800 steps	
2	15–20 minutes	451–650 steps	
1	9–15 minutes	400–450 steps	

6

CARDIOVASCULAR FITNESS

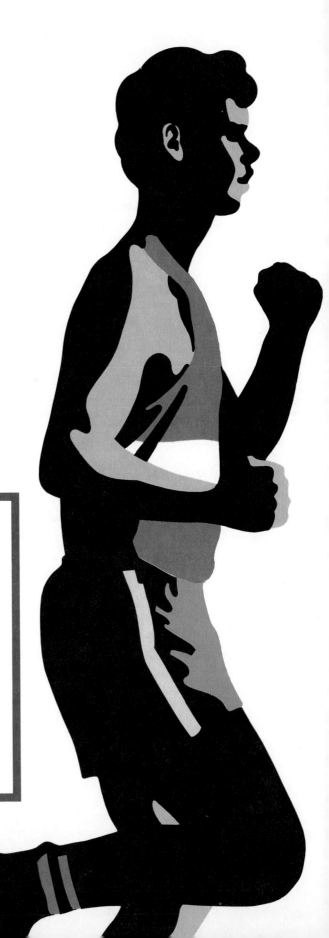

CHAPTER OBJECTIVES

After reading this chapter, you should be able to:

✔ Discuss the importance of cardio-vascular fitness.

✔ Explain how exercise helps reduce the risk of cardiovascular diseases.

✔ Explain how the FIT Formula can be applied to cardiovascular fitness.

✔ List activities that can help build cardiovascular fitness.

Cardiovascular fitness is fitness of the heart, lungs, blood, and blood vessels. "Cardio" is from the Greek word for heart; "vascular" refers to blood vessels. Of the eleven parts of fitness, cardiovascular fitness is the most important. It helps you increase your energy level, letting you be active for longer periods of time without tiring or getting out of breath. Cardiovascular fitness also helps you look good because it helps you control your weight and develop a good physique, or figure. In this chapter you will learn about your *cardiovascular system*—the body system that moves oxygen and nutrients to body cells and removes cell wastes. You will also learn how to improve your cardiovascular fitness.

CARDIOVASCULAR FITNESS AND GOOD HEALTH

To develop and maintain good health, you need to strengthen your heart muscle and also improve the other parts of your cardiovascular system. By exercising regularly, you will have a stronger heart muscle than a person who does very little exercise. You also increase the fitness of other parts of your cardiovascular system, such as the blood vessels and blood.

Scientific studies show that active people have less heart disease and are less likely to die from heart attacks than inactive people. Some symptoms of heart disease start to develop when people are in their teens. Therefore, it is important to develop and maintain cardiovascular fitness early in life.

EXERCISE AND BODY SYSTEMS

Regular exercise benefits two vital body systems—your cardiovascular system and your *respiratory system*—the body system that includes your lungs, brings oxygen to your bloodstream, and eliminates carbon dioxide from your bloodstream. The cardiovascular and respiratory systems work together to bring your body cells what they need to function and to rid the cells of wastes. Exercise helps these systems function more effectively and efficiently.

HEART Because your heart is a muscle, it benefits from exercise and activities, such as jogging, swimming, or hiking long distances. Your heart acts as a pump to supply blood to your body systems. Your *heart rate* is the number of times your heart beats per minute to pump blood through your body. Your *resting heart rate* is taken when you are relatively inactive. A person who exercises regularly might have a resting heart rate of 55 to 60 beats per minute, while a person who does not exercise regularly might have a resting heart rate of 70 or more beats per minute. A very fit person's heart beats approximately 9.5 million times less each year than that of the average person. Note in the picture how a fit person's heart pumps more blood with fewer beats, thus working more efficiently.

When you exercise vigorously, your muscles need more oxygen. Your heart pumps more blood to supply your muscles with more oxygen. Your heart has two ways to get more blood to your muscles: by beating faster or by sending a greater amount of blood with each beat. If your muscles do not get enough oxygen and their waste products are not removed, they cannot work effectively. As a result, the ability of your muscles to contract will be reduced; they will become tired. Obviously, your heart's ability to pump blood is very important when exercising, especially when exercising for an extended length of time.

LUNGS Your lungs must also be healthy to achieve good cardiovascular fitness. Your blood picks up oxygen in the lungs and carries it to the muscles. If your lungs are not healthy, your blood cannot pick up oxygen efficiently. Without enough oxygen, you will not be able to exercise vigorously for long periods of time. Because smoking causes direct damage to the lungs and other parts of the respiratory and cardiovascular systems, smoking is discouraged for people who want to have good cardiovascular fitness.

HAVE YOU HEARD?

The human heart is very efficient. It converts about one-half of its fuel into energy. A car is much less efficient. It converts only about 25 percent of its fuel into energy.

ARTERIES Your *arteries* are the "pipelines" that carry blood from your heart to other parts of your body. Blood is forced through the arteries by the beating of the heart.

A strong heart and healthy lungs are not very helpful if your arteries are not clear and open. Deposits inside an artery's walls thicken the walls, making the artery smaller and reducing blood flow. The buildup of deposits can lead to atherosclerosis—a disease in which the arteries become dangerously clogged and the deposits harden. An extreme case of atherosclerosis can totally block the blood flow in an artery. Also, the hardened deposits allow blood clots to form, severely blocking blood flow. In either case, the heart muscle does not get enough oxygen and a heart attack occurs. A heart attack's severity ranges from being barely noticeable to being fatal.

One of the causes of atherosclerosis and other cardiovascular diseases is too much of certain fats in the blood. Generally speaking, saturated fats and a fatty substance called cholesterol are potentially harmful to your cardiovascular system; unsaturated fats are not. *Saturated fats* are what most people commonly think of when they hear the word "fat." They include the fats in dairy products and the visible fat in red meat. *Cholesterol* is a fatty substance found in meats, dairy products, and egg yolks. *Unsaturated fats* are found in many kinds of oils, such as olive oil, peanut oil, corn oil, and sunflower oil. Chapter 12 discusses fats and other nutrients in more detail.

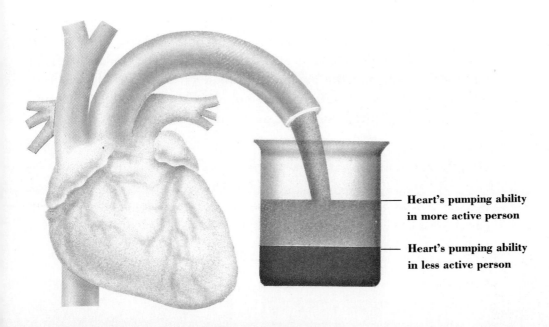

Heart's pumping ability in more active person

Heart's pumping ability in less active person

A strong heart can pump much more blood with each beat than a weaker heart can.

People in southern Italy have one of the lowest cardiovascular-disease rates in the world. Scientists attribute this to what is called the traditional Mediterranean diet, rich in fish, grains, fruits, vegetables, and olive oil.

Although your body needs a certain amount of fat and cholesterol, excessive amounts trigger formation of the fatty deposits along artery walls. Cholesterol can be especially dangerous partly because high levels can build in your body without you noticing it; even a thin person could have a high cholesterol level. Research has shown that cholesterol is carried through the bloodstream by particles called lipoproteins. One kind is *high-density lipoprotein* (HDL). HDL is often referred to as "good cholesterol" because HDLs carry excess cholesterol out of the bloodstream and into the liver for elimination from the body. Therefore, HDLs appear to help prevent atherosclerosis. However, *low-density lipoprotein* (LDL) is often referred to as "bad cholesterol" because LDLs carry cholesterol that is most likely to stay in the body and contribute to atherosclerosis.

Most people have a large degree of control over their cardiovascular fitness. The best approach is to cut down on dietary cholesterol and saturated fats and to get regular aerobic exercise. Cutting down on cholesterol and saturated fats helps reduce LDL levels in the blood. A healthful change in a person's eating habits does not have to be drastic. The American Heart Association recommends these guidelines:

- Select lean cuts of meat; trim off visible fat before cooking.
- Remove skin from poultry before cooking. Eat more fish.
- Avoid frying foods. Bake, steam, roast, boil, or broil foods.
- Drink low-fat or skim milk rather than whole milk.
- Use seasonings instead of butter and sauces to flavor food.
- Try fruit and plain cookies for desserts.
- Limit egg consumption to no more than three per week.

Regular exercise helps improve your cardiovascular fitness in several ways. First, it reduces LDL levels. Second, exercise is thought to increase HDL levels. Third, exercise can help prevent blood clots from forming by reducing the amount of fibrin in the blood. Fibrin is a substance involved in making the blood clot. Therefore, high amounts of fibrin might contribute to the development of atherosclerosis.

Regular exercise has still other benefits. How do the drawings of the two hearts on this page differ? Note that one has a richer network of blood vessels. Scientists have found that people who exercise regularly might develop more branching of the arteries in the heart. The importance of this richer network can be shown in this example. After astronaut Ed White died in a fire in 1967 while training for a mission, an autopsy was performed. The doctors found that one of the major arteries in his heart was completely blocked due to atherosclerosis. Because of all the physical training astronauts do, scientists believed White's body had developed an extra branching of arteries in his heart muscle. Therefore, he did not die of a heart attack when a main artery was blocked. White had been able to continue a high level of physical fitness training without signs of heart trouble.

VEINS Your *veins* carry blood filled with waste products from the muscle cells back to the heart. One-way valves in your veins help keep the blood from flowing backward. Your muscles squeeze the veins to pump the blood back to your heart. Regular exercise helps make your muscles squeeze your veins efficiently. A lack of exercise or movement can cause the valves, especially those in the legs, to stop working efficiently. Proper circulation in your legs is then reduced.

HAVE YOU HEARD?

In Chapter 3, you learned about cooling down after exercising. The squeezing action of your muscles on your veins during a cool-down is the reason your body recovers from exercise more effectively.

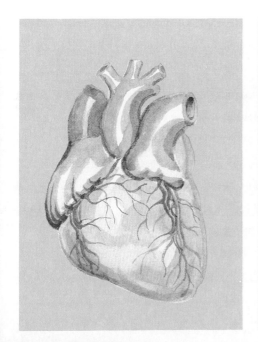

Normal circulation

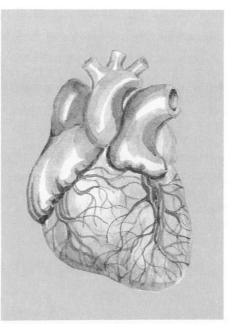

More branching of vessels from exercise

NERVES OF YOUR HEART Your heart muscle is not like your arm and leg muscles. To move your arm or leg, your muscles respond to a message sent by your brain. Muscles such as these respond when your brain tells them to do so. In contrast, your heart is not controlled voluntarily. It beats regularly without your having to tell it to beat. Nerves controlled by the brain automatically tell the heart to beat. Regular exercise can influence your nervous system to slow down your heart rate. In other words, regular exercise helps your heart work more efficiently. Each heartbeat supplies more blood and oxygen to your body than if you did not exercise. In addition, a person with a slower heart rate can function more effectively during an emergency or vigorous exercise.

The chart below summarizes the beneficial effects of exercise on the different parts of your cardiovascular system. In the following sections, you can learn how to achieve these benefits.

ACHIEVING CARDIOVASCULAR FITNESS

There are two major kinds of exercise: aerobic and anaerobic. Each can be performed to achieve cardiovascular fitness.

AEROBIC EXERCISE The term "aerobic" means "with oxygen." *Aerobic exercise* is exercise that is steady enough for the heart to supply all the oxygen your muscles need. Aerobic activities include jogging, walking, swimming, and bicycling at a slow, steady pace.

Benefits of Exercise on the Heart, Lungs, and Blood Vessels

Heart	• muscle gets bigger • pumps more blood per beat • beats fewer times per minute • works more efficiently
Lungs	• slower but deeper breathing while exercising • work more efficiently
Blood Vessels: Arteries	• less fat in the bloodstream • less risk of atherosclerosis • development of extra blood vessels • less risk of blood clot leading to heart attack
Veins	• stay healthy

ANAEROBIC EXERCISE The term "anaerobic" means "without oxygen." *Anaerobic exercise* is done in short, fast bursts. As a result, the heart cannot supply blood and oxygen to the muscles as fast as the muscles can use it. Without oxygen, you cannot exercise very long. You need frequent rests during anaerobic exercise to "catch your breath." Anaerobic activities include the 100-yard dash, 50-meter breaststroke, basketball, and handball.

FIT FORMULA AND CARDIOVASCULAR FITNESS

The best way to determine if an exercise contributes to cardiovascular fitness is to measure the increase in your heart rate during exercise. There are two target heart rates for cardiovascular fitness—one for aerobic exercise and the other for anaerobic exercise. This chart lists the minimum duration of exercise needed to develop cardiovascular fitness. More time is necessary if you want to improve other parts of fitness as well.

HAVE YOU HEARD?

Your heart can beat 200 times or more per minute when you exercise vigorously. As you grow older, your maximum heart rate decreases. By age 40, your heart will beat about 180 times per minute when it beats its fastest.

Fitness Target Zones for Cardiovascular Fitness

	Aerobic	Anaerobic
Frequency	Exercise at least 3 days a week. For best results, exercise 3 to 6 days a week.	Exercise at least 3 days a week. For best results, exercise every day.
Intensity	Raise your heart rate to your target heart rate zone.	Raise your heart rate to your target heart rate zone.
Time	Keep your heart rate in target zone for at least 15 minutes and for up to an hour.	Keep your heart rate in target zone for 10 to 40 seconds. Rest by walking or doing slow exercise for 3 times the length of the exercise. Total exercise time should be at least 15 minutes.

BUILDING CARDIOVASCULAR FITNESS

Each of these activities helps develop cardiovascular fitness. Other good activities for cardiovascular fitness include backpacking, cross-country skiing, soccer, wrestling, and rowing.

Pick a sport that has continuous activity and raises your heart rate, such as racquetball. Sports that require short bursts of exercise and long periods of rest are not as effective for cardiovascular fitness. If you choose a sport such as tennis, keep moving. Try to cut down on long waiting periods. Keep the tempo of the sport at an active level.

Remember to work above your minimum threshold of training and in your fitness target zone to improve your cardiovascular fitness. For example, if you jog, you should:

- Jog 3 to 6 days a week.
- Jog fast enough to raise your heart rate to the correct intensity.
- Jog at least 5 to 15 minutes, although 15 to 30 minutes is better.

JOGGING Use the correct jogging technique. Push off with the ball of your foot and land on the heel of your foot or on your entire foot. Wear well-made shoes with a cushioned heel and ample support. Use your heart rate to determine how much you should jog. No particular distance is best for all people.

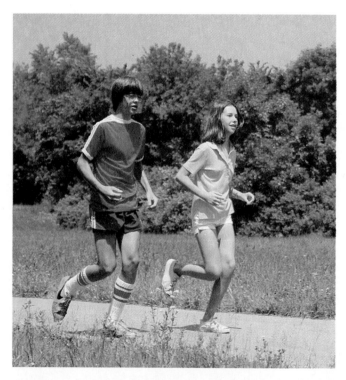

Jogging is an excellent cardiovascular activity.

WALKING Walk briskly enough to raise your heart rate to your minimum intensity level. If you walk with someone else, walk with someone of a similar cardiovascular fitness level. Keep in mind that walking uphill raises your heart rate more than walking on level ground.

SWIMMING The benefits of swimming depend on the stroke you are doing. The better you are at doing a stroke, the faster you must swim to raise your heart rate. Kicking your legs is as important as using your arms. Concentrate on using both arms and legs. Even poor swimmers can benefit from swimming. In fact, poor swimmers raise their heart rates higher than good swimmers.

Speed strokes, such as the crawl and butterfly, are anaerobic. For anaerobic swimming, swim fast sprints, then rest between sprints.

BICYCLING Bicycle at a steady pace; avoid coasting. Keep in mind that bicycling uphill raises your heart rate more than bicycling on level ground. For anaerobic bicycling, alternate bicycling fast and then resting by coasting or bicycling slowly.

AEROBIC DANCE Aerobic dance is a combination of dance steps and calisthenics done to music. Jackie Sorenson developed it as a way to exercise that was more fun than regular calisthenics and other aerobic exercise, such as jogging. Aerobic dance is done continuously, so it is a form of aerobic exercise. Dance routines are designed to elevate the person's heart rate to the target heart rate. Today, there are many forms of dance exercise similar to aerobic dance, such as rhythmic aerobics, step aerobics, and slimnastics. This chapter's *Focus on Fitness* features a sample aerobic dance routine.

CALISTHENICS Calisthenics must be done continuously to effectively build cardiovascular fitness. Exercise steadily and without interruption. If exercises are very active, jog in place between exercises.

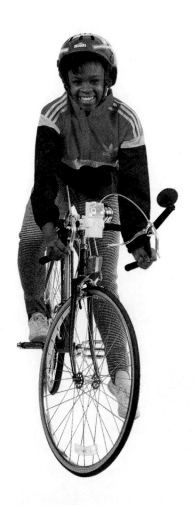

Bicycling is also a good cardiovascular activity.

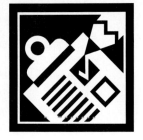

SELF-EVALUATION

CARDIOVASCULAR FITNESS

WORKSHEET 6-1

Use worksheet 6-1 to record and interpret the results of your self-evaluation.

Early in your exercise program, test yourself to see just how fit you are. After you have exercised regularly over a period of time, test yourself to see how much you have improved.

Lab tests are the most accurate way to measure cardiovascular fitness. They involve use of special equipment and are done in a physical-fitness laboratory. Lab tests are often done on a stationary bicycle or on a treadmill. These tests are sometimes called graded exercise tests, or stress tests, because they measure how your heart responds to vigorous exercise.

Most people do not live near a physical-fitness laboratory that has the equipment necessary to take an exercise stress test. To substitute, the 1-mile run, the 12-minute run, and the step test are used to measure cardiovascular fitness without special equipment. You can test yourself using one of the tests. You will need a place to run and a watch or clock with a second hand. You will also need a low bench or step if you take the step test.

ONE-MILE RUN Take the 1-mile run test for your own information. Do your best, but keep in mind that individuals' abilities differ; this is not a race. Your goal is a "good fitness" rating. Once you achieve a "good fitness" score, a faster time does not necessarily improve your health. However, it might help you perform better in a sport or other activity. *Note:* Exercise for several days a week for several weeks before you take this test.

As you take the test, try to set a pace that you can keep up for the full mile. A steady pace is best. If you start too fast and then have to slow down at the end, you will probably not be able to run as fast for the entire distance.

1. Run or jog for 1 mile in the shortest time possible. Your score is the amount of time it takes you to run the mile.

2. Find your rating on the cardiovascular fitness rating chart. The chart is on page 72.

TWELVE-MINUTE RUN Follow the same directions as for the 1-mile run, only run as far as you can in 12 minutes. Your score is the distance you cover in 12 minutes (measured to the nearest 20 yards). Use the cardiovascular fitness rating chart to determine your rating. The chart is on page 72.

THE STEP TEST To do this test, step up and down on a 12-inch high bench for 3 minutes. *Note:* Exercise several days a week for several weeks before you take this test.
1. Step up with your right foot. Step up with your left foot.
2. Step down with your right foot. Step down with your left foot. Repeat this 4-count (up, up, down, down); step 24 times each minute.
3. Immediately after stepping for 3 minutes, sit down and count your own neck pulse or have a partner count your neck pulse. Begin counting within 5 seconds after you stop stepping. Count for 1 minute.
4. Record your results on your worksheet. You are only expected to do this test once in class unless your instructor tells you otherwise. Check your cardiovascular rating and write it on your worksheet. The chart is on page 72.

HAVE YOU HEARD?

Cardiovascular fitness can be measured using a PACER (Progressive Aerobic Cardiovascular Endurance Run) test. To do this test, a person runs 20 meters several times in a row. Each run is progressively faster. Final score is the number of runs a person can do while still keeping up with the pace.

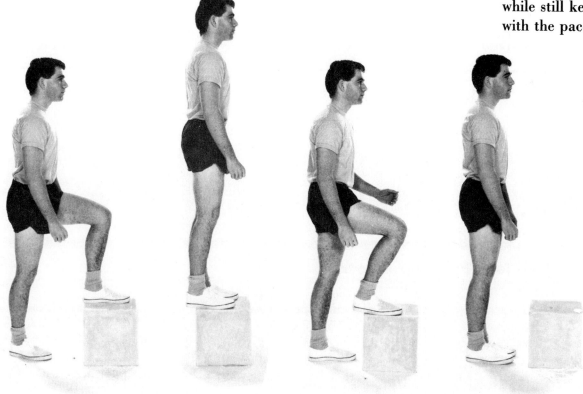

Rating Charts: Cardiovascular Fitness

One Mile Run *(time in minutes and seconds)*

Age		Good Performance	Good Fitness	Marginal Fitness	Low Fitness
13 years or less	males	7:30 or less	7:31–9:00	9:01–9:56	over 10:00
	females	7:30 or less	7:31–9:00	11:01–12:29	over 12:30
14–16 years	males	7:30 or less	7:01–8:00	8:01–9:29	over 9:30
	females	9:15 or less	9:16–10:30	10:31–11:59	over 12:00
17 years or more	males	6:40 or less	6:34–8:00	8:01–8:59	over 9:00
	females	9:15 or less	9:16–10:30	10:31–11:59	over 12:00

12 Minute Run *(distance in yards)*

Age		Good Performance	Good Fitness	Marginal Fitness	Low Fitness
13 years or less	males	over 2650	2500–2649	2400–2499	2399 or less
	females	over 1900	1800–1899	1700–1799	1699 or less
14–16 years	males	over 2800	2600–2799	2500–2599	2799 or less
	females	over 2100	1900–2099	1700–1899	1699 or less
17 years or more	males	over 3000	2800–2999	2600–2799	2599 or less
	females	over 2300	2000–2299	1700–1999	1699 or less

Step Test *(beats per minute)*

Age		Good Performance	Good Fitness	Marginal Fitness	Low Fitness
13 years or less	males	90 or less	91–98	99–120	above 120
	females	100 or less	101–110	111–130	above 130
14–16 years	males	85 or less	86–95	96–115	above 115
	females	95 or less	96–105	106–125	above 125
17 years or more	males	80 or less	81–90	91–110	above 110
	females	90 or less	91–100	101–120	above 120 (or those who cannot step 3 minutes)

CHAPTER REVIEW

MULTIPLE CHOICE

Choose the letter of the best answer.

1. Cardiovascular fitness includes fitness of your (a) skin. (b) respiratory system. (c) excretory system (d) digestive system.

2. A fit person's heart works efficiently because it (a) pumps more blood with relatively fewer beats. (b) beats more often than an unfit person's heart. (c) is generally smaller than an unfit person's heart. (d) beats less often and pumps less blood with each beat.

3. Which system works with your cardiovascular system to bring nutrients to body cells? (a) muscular system (b) excretory system (c) respiratory system (d) digestive system

4. A heart attack can occur when (a) a certain virus infects the bloodstream. (b) a blood vessel bursts. (c) the heart does not get enough carbon dioxide. (d) an artery in the heart becomes blocked.

5. Which is an example of aerobic exercise? (a) walking (b) sprinting (c) baseball (d) raquetball

6. Regular exercise helps improve cardiovascular fitness by (a) reducing HDL levels. (b) reducing LDL levels. (c) producing cholesterol. (d) producing fibrin.

7. Which substance is the least harmful to your cardiovascular system? (a) low-density lipoprotein (b) high-density lipoprotein (c) unsaturated fats (d) cholesterol

8. In the FIT Formula, "intensity" refers to (a) how often you exercise. (b) how long you exercise. (c) how hard you exercise. (d) the kind of exercise you do.

9. Exercise to improve cardiovascular fitness at least (a) twice a day. (b) twice a week. (c) five times a week. (d) three times a week.

10. Exercise improves cardiovascular fitness only if the exercise (a) is anaerobic. (b) raises your heart rate as much as possible. (c) raises your heart rate to your correct intensity level. (d) is aerobic.

MATCHING

Match the definition in Column I with the term it defines in Column II.

Column I

11. carry blood away from the heart
12. fatty substance in meats and egg yolks
13. found in many oils, such as corn oil
14. carries excess cholesterol out of the body
15. exercise done in short bursts

Column II

a. anaerobic exercise
b. arteries
c. cholesterol
d. high-density lipoprotein
e. unsaturated fats

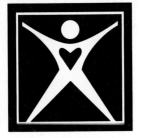

FOCUS ON FITNESS

AEROBIC DANCE

Aerobic dance—a popular form of exercise—is a dance routine that is also a form of aerobic exercise. Practice each dance step shown here. The chart combines the dance steps into a dance routine. Perform the routine to music that has a strong four-count rhythm. If you make a mistake or lose your place, keep moving. Catch up when you can. Remember to warm up before and cool down afterwards.

AEROBIC DANCE ROUTINE

Counts	Step	Repetitions	Counts	Step	Repetitions
16	Stand and clap to the music		8	Backward Jog	4 steps with each foot
			8	Jumping Jack	4 times
32	Step/Hop	4 times (8 counts per repetition)	32	Jesse Polka	4 left and 4 right
			16	Grapevine	2 times
8	Forward Jog	4 steps with each foot	16	High Kicks	4 left and 4 right
8	Jumping Jack	4 times	16	Step/Hop	4 times

STEP HOP Follow the directions below. After you have learned the step, clap your hands on every fourth count (with the hop-kick).
- On 1, step with your right foot.
- On 2, step with your left foot.
- On 3, step with your right foot.
- On 4, hop on your right foot and kick with your left leg.
- Repeat counts 1 through 4, but start with your left foot.

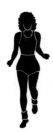 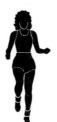 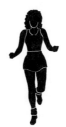 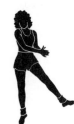

FORWARD JOG Jog forward to the beat of the music. Take short steps, especially when in a small space.

JUMPING JACK Follow these directions:
- On 1, jump and spread your feet shoulder width and bring both arms over your head.
- On 2, jump and bring your feet together. Bring arms to sides.

BACKWARD JOG Jog backward to the beat of the music. Take short steps equal to those done in the forward jog.

JESSE POLKA STEP Follow these directions:
- On 1, hop on your left leg and kick with your right leg.
- On 2, hop on your left leg and kick your right heel in front of your left leg.
- On 3, hop on your left leg and kick with your right leg.
- On 4, bring both feet together.
- Repeat counts 1 through 4, but start with your right foot. Raise your arms on counts 1 and 3, and lower them on counts 2 and 4.

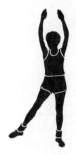 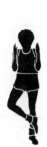 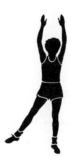 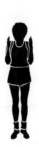

GRAPEVINE Follow these directions:
- On 1, step to your left with your left foot.
- On 2, step across in front of your left foot with your right foot.
- On 3, step to the left with your left foot.
- On 4, kick your right foot in front of your left leg as you hop on your left foot. You might also clap on this count.
- Repeat counts 1 through 4, but start with your right foot.

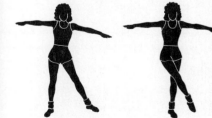 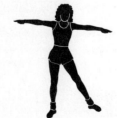 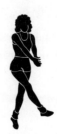

HIGH KICK Follow these directions:
- On 1, hop on your right foot as you kick with your left foot.
- On 2, hop on your left foot as you kick with your right foot.

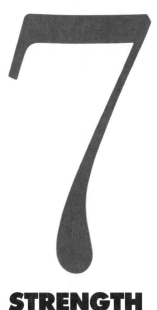

7

STRENGTH

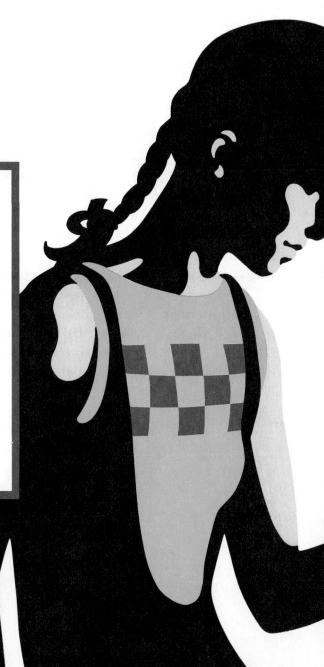

CHAPTER OBJECTIVES

After reading this chapter, you should be able to:

✔ Explain the importance of strength.

✔ Distinguish between isotonic and isometric exercises.

✔ Apply the FIT Formula to strength.

✔ Recognize some misconceptions about strength training.

✔ Recall safety precautions to follow when weight training or performing isometric exercises.

Strength is the amount of force a muscle can exert. Strong muscles can help you jump, lift, push, pull, carry, and do other activities more easily. You need strength to move heavy loads and for some emergencies—perhaps to save your own or someone else's life in a fire or an accident. If your muscles regularly work against heavy loads, they will stay strong. If you do not use your muscles, they become weak. In this chapter you will learn about the importance of strength and how you can strengthen your body with regular exercise.

TYPES OF MUSCLES

Each of your body's three types of muscles have specific functions. *Smooth muscles* make up the walls of hollow internal organs such as the stomach and blood vessels. Your heart is made of *cardiac muscle*. Both smooth and cardiac muscles are called *involuntary muscles* because you do not consciously control their movements.

Skeletal muscles are attached to bones and make movement possible. These muscles are called *voluntary muscles* because you can control their movements. You control your voluntary muscles when you decide to walk, run, lift or hold an object, or perform other actions.

STRENGTH AND GOOD HEALTH

Strong muscles help you to maintain good posture and are necessary to participate in certain sports and exercises. Strength can also help reduce fatigue, and help prevent muscle injuries and muscle soreness. Injury and soreness most likely occur when a person exercises vigorously after having been inactive for long periods of time. If your muscles are strong, you are more able to withstand vigorous activity.

Muscular strength can prevent some health problems. Strong back and abdominal muscles can help prevent backache. More adults see their doctor for back pain than for almost any other medical problem.

STRENGTH FOR MALES AND FEMALES Every person should have enough strength to maintain good health. Active people who do a lot of lifting need more strength than people who are not as active. The amount of strength you need to stay healthy and to do what you want depends upon your own personal needs and interests.

Some people think that only men and boys need to be concerned with their strength. This idea is not true. Both males and females need strength to be healthy, to avoid injury, and to look good. Usually, the hormones in females' bodies prevent them from developing large, bulky muscles even when they exercise regularly. However, women and girls who perform strength exercises do develop strong muscles. Both men and women look more attractive with strong muscles.

FITNESS PRINCIPLES AND STRENGTH

The three basic fitness principles can be applied to strength exercises. You read about these principles—overload, progression, and specificity—in Chapter 4.

PRINCIPLE OF OVERLOAD A muscle must contract harder than normal if it is to become stronger. In other words, the muscle must work more than normal. If a muscle is worked less than normal, it will weaken. If a muscle is always worked against the same amount of resistance, it will maintain the same strength. Your muscles eventually adapt to the load, so it feels easy to move. When it begins to feel easy, increase the load.

PRINCIPLE OF PROGRESSION Overload gradually—increase the load over a period of time—to get the best improvement in muscle strength. You can injure yourself if you try to lift too much weight too soon. Also, lifting too much weight too soon will not result in as much strength gain as would occur if you progressed gradually.

PRINCIPLE OF SPECIFICITY You must exercise the specific muscles you expect to develop. For example, leg exercises develop the legs; arm exercises develop the arms. This principle also means you should do some strength exercises that closely resemble the movement that you want to eventually use.

HOW STRONG ARE YOU? Before starting an exercise program to build muscle strength, test yourself to see just how fit you are. Once you have evaluated yourself, you can exercise to improve your strength. After you have been exercising for a while, test yourself again to see how much you have improved.

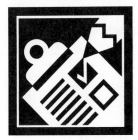

SELF-EVALUATION

STRENGTH

PART 1: BODY WEIGHT STRENGTH A good way to evaluate your strength is to see if you can handle your own body weight. Handling your own body weight includes being able to lift yourself, handle yourself if you should fall, and carry your own body effectively. Some experts think that how much you can lift might not be nearly as important as whether you can handle your own body weight when necessary.

Use part 1 to determine if you have enough strength to handle your own body weight. If you cannot do each exercise, you might start an exercise program to improve your strength. Follow these directions:
1. If possible, complete the number of repetitions specified.
2. Record on your worksheet the number of times you did each exercise. Use only the "First Test" column on the worksheet. You are expected to do this test only once in class unless your instructor tells you otherwise. Use the rest of the worksheet for future tests.
3. Find your rating on the rating chart. Record it on your worksheet.

WORKSHEET 7-1

Use worksheet 7-1 to record and interpret your results of this self-evalution.

Rating Chart: Body Weight Strength

Rating	Number of tests passed
Good	4
Marginal	3
Low	less than 3

TRUNK CURL

1. Lie on your back; arms extended, palms on the floor.
2. Bend your knees at a 90° angle.
3. Roll head and shoulders forward and upward enough to lift shoulder blades off the floor. The tips of your fingers will slide forward. *Caution:* Do not lift your back off the floor.
4. Return to the starting position. Repeat 8 times.

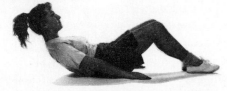

KNEE DIP

• This exercise tests your leg muscles. See page 160 for directions. Males should complete 8 repetitions with each leg to pass. Females should complete 5 repetitions with each leg to pass.

PULL-UP

• This exercise tests your arm and shoulder muscles.
1. Hang from a bar with your arms straight and your palms facing away from your body. Keep your feet off the ground.
2. Pull until your chin is even with the bar. Lower yourself to the starting position. Males should complete 2 repetitions to pass. Females should be able to pull up until the upper arm is parallel to the bar.

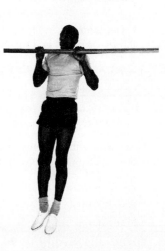

HALF PUSH-UP

● This exercise tests your arm muscles.
1. Lie face down, hands on the floor next to your shoulders.
2. Keep your body straight. Push up until your upper arms are parallel to the floor.

3. Lower your body until your nose touches the floor. Only your toes and hands may touch the floor. Males should complete 8 repetitions to pass. Females should complete 6 repetitions to pass.

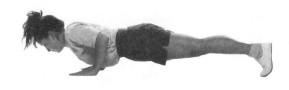

PART 2: GRIP AND LEG STRENGTH A dynamometer test is also a good test of strength. If one is available, use this device to test the strength of several muscle groups. Part 2 tests your grip strength and your hip and leg strength. In class, you might only have time to take the tests once. However, retest yourself periodically, if possible.

GRIP STRENGTH

1. If your dynamometer is adjustable, adjust it to fit your hand.
2. Squeeze the grip dynamometer as hard as you can. Then read your score on the dynamometer dial. Do the test twice with each hand. Use the better of the two scores.

3. Record your scores on your worksheet. Find your rating in the rating chart. Record your right- and left-hand ratings on your worksheet.

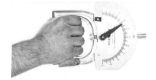

LEG STRENGTH

1. Hold the handle of the leg dynamometer while the instructor adjusts it to fit you.
2. Pull up on the handle by trying to straighten your legs while keeping your back and arms straight.
3. When you have finished pulling, the

instructor will read your score on the dynamometer dial. Record your score on your worksheet. Then find your rating in the rating chart. Record your rating on your worksheet.

Rating Chart: Grip Strength and Leg Strength

Strength in Kilograms

Grip Strength Fitness Rating	Below 15 years old males right	left	females right	left	15 to 17 years old males right	left	females right	left	18 years and over males right	left	females right	left
Performance	50	47	35	30	60	57	38	35	70	68	40	37
Good Fitness	45	42	30	25	53	50	32	30	60	55	40	36
Marginal	37	35	25	20	45	42	27	25	50	45	28	25
Low Fitness	32	30	20	18	40	35	20	18	45	40	20	18

Leg Strength Fitness Rating	Below 15 years old males	females	15 to 17 years old males	females	18 years and over males	females
Performance	177	100	206	116	240	135
Good Fitness	155	82	180	95	210	110
Marginal	116	48	135	56	155	65
Low Fitness	103	37	120	43	140	50

IMPROVING MUSCLE STRENGTH

You must exert muscular force against a resistance to improve muscle strength. Both isotonic and isometric exercises help improve muscle strength. *Isotonic exercises* are those in which muscles shorten or lengthen as they contract and body parts move. Isotonic exercises are usually done by lifting weights or by doing calisthenics.

Isometric exercises are those in which the muscles contract when working against a stationary object or body part that is prevented from moving. The muscles work, but the body parts do not move.

WHICH TYPE IS BETTER? Both isotonic and isometric exercise help build strength. Some experts feel that isotonic exercise is the better form of exercise because it develops more strength than isometric exercise. However, isotonic exercise often requires special equipment to provide an overload.

Isometric exercises do not require equipment and can be done in a small area. Since you should train the way you are going to use your muscles, isometrics are useful preparation if you frequently lift and carry heavy objects. However, isometric exercises also have disadvantages. You have no way of knowing if you are working as hard as you should. Also, isometric muscle contractions significantly increase blood pressure; persons with high blood pressure should probably avoid isometric exercises.

MUSCLE-BOUND A mistaken belief about strength exercises is that they can cause a person to have tight, bulky muscles that prevent them from moving freely. Such a condition is often referred to as being *muscle-bound.* Usually people become muscle-bound either because they have not exercised correctly or because they developed a few muscles while neglecting others.

When lifting weights, be sure to move your joints through their full range of motion. For example, your elbow joint can bend to allow your hand to reach your shoulder and to let your arm straighten completely. Therefore, in weight training, bend your elbow all the way to lift the weight, as shown here. Straighten it as you lower the weight. *Caution:* Do not bend your elbow or other joint backwards beyond a full range of motion. You can damage your joint.

STEROIDS Some people take *anabolic steroids* to make themselves stronger or to make their muscles more bulky. This practice is extremely dangerous since steroids can damage the liver and even cause cancer of the liver. Also, anabolic steroids can cause rapid weight gain, acne, stunted growth, and aggressive behavior. Other conditions, such as high blood pressure, premature coronary artery disease, and sterility have been linked to anabolic steroid use.

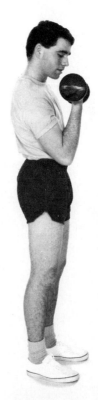

Moving the elbow joint through its full range of motion.

THE FIT FORMULA AND STRENGTH

You already know that the only way to strengthen your muscles is to make them work against greater loads than normal, or overload them. Exercise in your *target zone* to achieve the best results from strength exercises. This fitness target zone chart shows the amount of exercise needed to improve muscle strength. This program starts with 5 repetitions and increases to 8 repetitions. Other weight-training programs use different durations; some people combine both isotonic and isometric programs. Programs such as these are also effective.

REPETITIONS AND SETS Every other day, work to complete 3 sets of 5 to 8 repetitions of each exercise for both isotonic weight training and isotonic calisthenics. *Repetitions* are the number of consecutive times you do each exercise. For example, if you repeat an exercise 5 times without stopping, you have completed 5 repetitions. Repetitions are sometimes referred to as "reps." A *set* is one group of repetitions. Repeat an exercise 5 times, then rest. Repeat it 5 times again, then rest. Finally, repeat the exercise another 5 times. You will have completed a total of 3 sets of 5 repetitions.

CORRECT INTENSITY This chart shows that you should lift heavy weights or contract your muscles as hard as you can to build strength. If you are doing isotonic exercises, lift the heaviest weights possible for the muscles you are exercising. You can use one of several methods to do so. For some people, just lifting the parts of the body, such as the arms and the legs, is enough. For others, lifting the entire body, as in a pull-up, might be necessary. For strong people, it might be necessary to lift extra weight to overload the muscles enough to develop strength. If you are doing isometric exercises, make your muscles contract as hard as you can for each exercise.

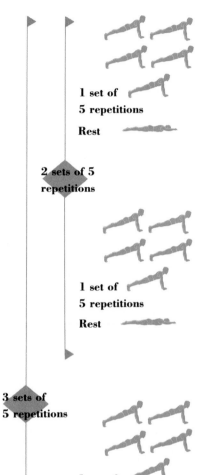

1 set of
5 repetitions

Rest

2 sets of 5
repetitions

1 set of
5 repetitions

Rest

3 sets of
5 repetitions

1 set of
5 repetitions

Fitness Target Zones for Strength

	Isotonic	Isometric
Frequency	Every other day and at least 3 days a week.	Every other day and at least 3 days a week.
Intensity	Move the heaviest weight you can lift for the required number of times.	Contract the muscles as tightly as possible for the required length of time.
Time	Begin with 3 sets of 5 repetitions. Gradually increase repetitions to 8. Rest 1 minute between sets.	Hold the contraction for 5 seconds. Complete 3 repetitions. Gradually increase to 8 seconds. Rest 30 seconds between contractions.

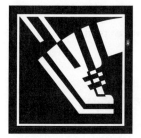

ACTIVITY

CALISTHENICS

Calisthenics help develop muscle strength. Examples include the exercises you completed in the self-evaluation for body weight strength as well as these exercises. Try the calisthenics described here. Choose a level based upon what you think you can do. The information you obtained about your own strength in the self-evaluation can help you choose. Keep these guidelines in mind:

• Perform an exercise for 3 sets of 5 to 8 repetitions in order to build strength. If you can complete 3 sets of 5 to 8 repetitions, but no more, then the exercise is just enough to help you build strength. When you can easily complete 3 sets of 8 repetitions, then you need to make the exercise harder. If you can do more than 8 repetitions in each set, then you are not "overloaded" enough to achieve best results.

• If you cannot complete 3 sets of 5 repetitions, then try a lower level. If you can do more than 3 sets of 5 repetitions, then try a higher level.

• Be careful when using extra weight. Have your instructor or a partner help you perform each exercise safely.

• Do strength-training exercises slowly; build up gradually. You will benefit more from the exercises.

WORKSHEET 7-2
Use worksheet 7-2 to record your results for this activity.

PULL-UP Pull-ups develop arm and shoulder muscles.

BEGINNING: PULL-UP WITH ASSISTANCE

• Do these pull-ups if you cannot complete 3 sets of 5 pull-ups.
1. Hang from a bar. Your palms face away from your body. Your feet are off the ground.
2. Have a partner give you a slight boost while you pull up until your chin is above the bar.
3. Slowly lower to starting position. Do 3 sets of 5 to 8 repetitions.

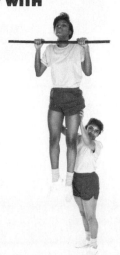

INTERMEDIATE: PULL-UP

• Do these pull-ups if you can complete at least 3 sets of 5 repetitions, but not 3 sets of 8 repetitions. See page 79 for directions. Do 3 sets of 5 to 8 repetitions.

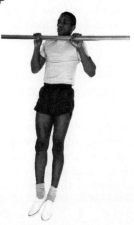

ADVANCED: PULL-UP WITH WEIGHT

● Do pull-ups with
weight if you can do 3
sets of 8 pull-ups.

1. Use two plastic milk
or bleach bottles with
caps and a short piece
of rope (24 to 36
inches). Tie one bottle
to each end of the rope.
2. Fill the bottles with
equal amounts of water
or sand. Put in only
enough water so that it
is hard for you to do 3
sets of 5 repetitions.
3. Hang the bottles
around your shoulders
so they hang in front of
you. You might put a
towel behind your neck
as a cushion.
4. Use the same weight
until you can do 3 sets
of 8 repetitions. Then
add more water or sand
to the bottles.

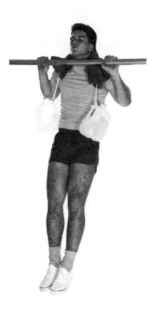

TRUNK CURL Trunk curls help strengthen
abdominal and hip flexor muscles.

BEGINNING: CURL

● Do these curls if you
cannot complete 3 sets
of 5 repetitions. See
page 18 for directions.

INTERMEDIATE: CURL WITH HANDS ON CHEEKS

● Do this exercise if you
can complete at least 3
sets of 5 repetitions, but
not 3 sets of 8 repetitions. See page 18 for
directions.

ADVANCED: CURL ON TILT BOARD

● Do this exercise if you
can complete 3 sets of 8
repetitions of curls with
your hands on your
cheeks. This exercise is
the same as the curl
except that you lie on a
tilt board with your feet
elevated about 18 inches
above your head. *Caution:* Do not let your
back leave the board.

PUSH-UP Push-ups develop arm and
chest muscles.

BEGINNING: BENT-KNEE PUSH-UP

● Do bent-knee push-
ups if you cannot com-
plete at least 3 sets of 5
push-ups. See page 21
for directions.

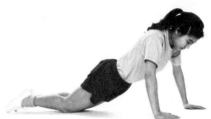

INTERMEDIATE: HALF PUSH-UP

● Do these push-ups if
you can complete at
least 3 sets of 5 repeti-
tions, but not 3 sets of 8
repetitions. See page 80
for directions.

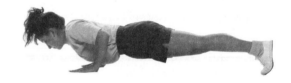

ADVANCED: PUSH-UP

● Do these push-ups if
you can complete 3 sets
of 8 repetitions of intermediate push-ups.
Complete 3 sets of 5 to 8
repetitions.

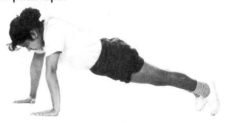

SQUAT AND KNEE DIP Squats and knee dips develop leg muscles.

BEGINNING: TWO-LEG SQUAT

• Do these squats if you cannot complete 3 sets of 5 repetitions.
1. Stand with your feet about 12 inches apart. Squat until your knees are bent at a 90° angle. Balance with your arms.
2. Return to standing position. Complete 3 sets of 5 to 8 repetitions.

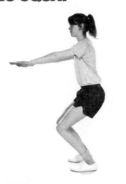

INTERMEDIATE: KNEE DIP

• Do knee dips if you can complete at least 3 sets of 5 repetitons, but not 3 sets of 8 repetitions. See page 160 for directions.

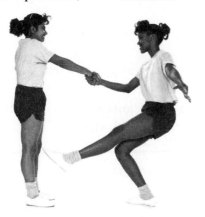

ADVANCED: KNEE DIP WITH WEIGHT

• Do this knee dip if you can complete 3 sets of 8 repetitions of knee dips. See page 102 for directions on how to make plastic-bottle weights. Hang the bottles around your shoulders and use a towel to cushion your neck. Try to complete 3 sets of 5 repetitions. Increase the repetitions until you can complete 3 sets of 8 repetitions using the same weight. Then increase the amount of water or sand in the bottles.

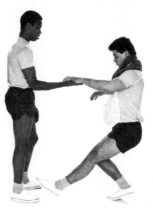

TENNIS BALL SQUEEZE Tennis ball squeezes develop grip strength. *Note:* This exercise is isotonic if you can squeeze hard enough to indent the ball. If you cannot indent the ball, the exercise is isometric.

BEGINNING: OLD BALL SQUEEZE

• Do this squeeze if you cannot complete 3 sets of 5 repetitions using a slightly-used tennis ball.
1. Hold an old tennis ball in your hand. Squeeze it as hard as you can.
2. Complete 3 sets of 5 to 8 repetitions if you are doing isotonic exercises. If you are doing isometric exercises, squeeze and hold the ball for 5 seconds, and then rest 30 seconds. Complete 3 repetitions.

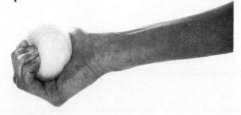

INTERMEDIATE: SLIGHTLY-USED BALL SQUEEZE

• Do these squeezes if you can complete 3 sets of 5 repetitions using a slightly-used tennis ball, but cannot complete 3 sets of 8 repetitions. Follow the same directions as above.

ADVANCED: NEW BALL SQUEEZE

• Do these squeezes if you can complete 3 sets of 8 repetitions using a slightly-used tennis ball. Follow the same directions as for the old ball squeeze.

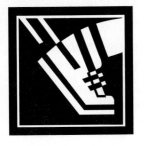

ACTIVITY

ISOMETRIC EXERCISES

You already know that isometric exercises help develop muscle strength. You can use your own body, a wall, or a rope as immovable resistance when performing isometric exercises. This activity includes examples of isometric exercises good for strengthening muscles.

Before beginning an isometric exercise program, be aware of these guidelines:

● People with high blood pressure probably should avoid isometric exercises.

● Never hold your breath while performing isometric exercises. You could black out.

● Be sure you are in your target zone. Contract your muscles as hard as you can and hold for 5 to 8 seconds each time.

WORKSHEET 7-3

Use worksheet 7-3 to record your results of this activity.

BACK FLATTENER

● This exercise helps develop your abdominal muscles.
1. Lie on your back with your knees bent.
2. Pull in your abdomen by contracting your abdominal muscles as tightly as possible. Flatten your lower back firmly against the floor. Hold for 5 seconds; rest 30 seconds.
3. Repeat 2 more times.

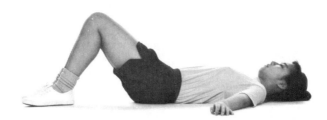

HAND PUSH

● This exercise helps develop your upper body and arms.
1. Sit on the floor with your back straight. You may cross your legs if you prefer. Clasp the palms of your hands together.

2. Raise your hands and elbows to shoulder height. Push your hands against each other as hard as you can. Hold for 5 seconds; rest 30 seconds.
3. Repeat 2 more times.

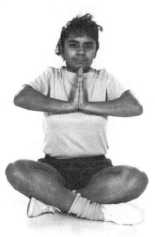

WALL PUSH

● This exercise helps develops your abdominal muscles and legs.
1. Stand with your back against a wall.
2. Move your feet out as you lower yourself into a half squat. Keep your thighs parallel to the floor.
3. Push your back against the wall by pushing with your legs as hard as you can. Hold for 5 seconds; rest 30 seconds.
4. Repeat 2 more times.

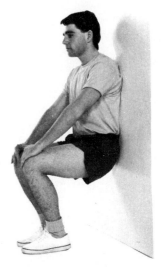

BICEPS CURL WITH ROPE

● This exercise helps develop your upper body and arms.
1. Stand with good posture. Loop a length of rope under your feet.
2. Grasp the rope ends with your palms up. Keep your elbows against your sides.
3. Pull up on the rope as hard as possible. Hold for 5 seconds; rest 30 seconds.
4. Repeat 2 more times.

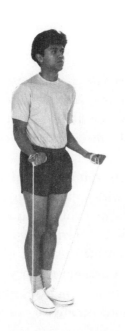

TOE PUSH

● This exercise helps develop your arms and lower legs.
1. Sit on the floor with good posture.
2. Hold the end of a rope in each hand. Loop it over your feet so it is tight against the soles of your feet.
3. Push forward with your feet as you pull on the rope. Keep back straight. Hold for 5 seconds; rest 30 seconds.
4. Repeat 2 more times.

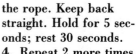
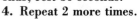
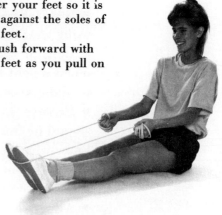

WEIGHT TRAINING

When done properly, weight training is one of the most effective kinds of strength exercises. Some people call weight training "pumping iron." Weight training can be done with free weights, weight machines, or homemade weights such as those made with plastic bottles filled with water or sand.

If your school has weight-training equipment, ask your instructor for more information about using it. For many people, isotonic calisthenics are enough to build as much strength as they want. However, if you choose to do weight training, do at least one exercise for each major muscle group in your body. For example, the bench press helps develop the muscles on the backs of your arms (triceps) and your chest muscles (pectorals). Half squats help develop your thigh muscles (quadriceps and hamstrings) and buttocks muscles (gluteals).

Weight-training machines are considered to be safer than free weights. There is a higher risk of injury when working with free weights unless you practice correctly and safely. Studies have shown that half of all people who are injured in weight training are between the ages of 10 and 19. Most of those injuries occurred while they were lifting weights at home. At the end of this chapter, a sample circuit weight-training program is presented. You might try it if the equipment is available. Your instructor could modify the machine exercise so that the same circuit could be performed with free weights.

Weight training is safest for people who have completed most of their growing. Consult with your instructor and your doctor if you are in doubt about weight training. Boys and girls who have not yet reached puberty, or who are going through puberty, should only weight train with close supervision.

WEIGHT-TRAINING CAUTIONS Keep these guidelines in mind when using weight-training machines, free weights, or homemade weights:
- Consult with your instructor about which exercises to do and how much weight to use. Not all exercises are good for everyone; some can be dangerous.
- Be sure the equipment fits you and is safe. Weight training can and should be fun, but playing with weights can be dangerous. Be sure you know what you are doing before you begin a weight-training program.
- Never compete when you do strength training. For example, do not have contests to see who can lift the most weight.
- Always use a "spotter" (partner) when you use free weights.
- When using a weight-training machine, start with one set and minimum weight so you can concentrate on correct technique and safety.

CHAPTER REVIEW

MULTIPLE CHOICE

Choose the letter of the best answer.

1. *Strength* refers to (a) the strain a muscle bears. (b) exercise done regularly. (c) the force a muscle can exert. (d) overload.
2. Which is best for developing strength? (a) isotonic exercise (b) leg exercises only (c) stretching exercises exercises only (d) long-distance running
3. Which type of muscles make movement possible? (a) smooth muscles (b) skeletal muscles (c) rough muscles (d) cardiac muscles
4. How many sets of each exercise should you do to build muscle strength? (a) 8 (b) 2 (c) 3 (d) 5
5. How often should weight training be done? (a) every day (b) twice a week (c) once a week (d) every other day
6. A set refers to (a) the amount of weight you can lift. (b) one group of repetitions. (c) degree to which you move an arm. (d) number of days per week you exercise.
7. An isometric exercise should be held (a) for 5 seconds each. (b) for 1 minute each. (c) for 30 seconds each. (d) as long as you can possibly hold it.
8. When you first start weight training, you should do one exercise (a) for each major muscle group. (b) at least 3 minutes. (c) every day. (d) as long as you can.
9. Which calisthenic is especially good for strengthening abdominal muscles? (a) push-up (b) squat and knee dip (c) stride step (d) trunk curl
10. Weight training is a(n) (a) isotonic exercise. (b) isometric exercise. (c) skill-building exercise. (d) flexibility exercise.

MATCHING

Match the definition in Column I with the term it defines in Column II.

Column I

11. can control their movements
12. cannot consciously control their movements
13. tight, bulky muscles
14. muscles lengthen or contract; body parts move
15. muscles contract; body parts do not move

Column II

a. involuntary muscles
b. isometric exercises
c. isotonic exercises
d. muscle-bound
e. voluntary muscles

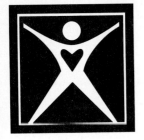

FOCUS ON FITNESS

WEIGHT TRAINING

Most weight machines provide stations to exercise muscle groups and let you set the amount of resistance you are working against. The exercises are selected so that most, but not all, major muscle groups are used and you do not use the same muscles consecutively. Follow these steps to determine how much weight you can lift:

1. Experiment to determine the amount of weight at each station that you can lift 5 times and no more. Write this weight down; it is your 5RM. (RM stands for **Repetitions: Maximum.**)

2. Calculate half of your 5RM. Write it down. It is your 1/2 5RM.

3. Calculate three-fourths of your 5RM and write it down. It is your 3/4 5RM. For example, if you can lift 50 pounds 5 times, that is your 5 RM. Thus, 1/2 5RM is 25 pounds; 3/4 5RM is about 37 pounds.

Follow this procedure for weight training. Remember to warm-up and stretch before exercising and to cool-down and stretch afterwards.

1. Perform the exercise at each station, doing 5 repetitions of 1/2 5RM. Rotate in the order in which the stations are listed.

2. When you have completed the stations, you have completed one set. Complete a second set, using 5 repetitions of 3/4 5RM.

3. Complete a third set, completing 5 repetitions of full 5RM.

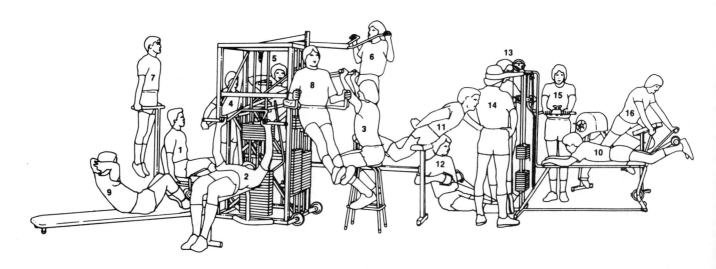

- **Leg Press (1)** Push the pedal, extending your hips and knees, to strengthen your thigh muscles (quadriceps). *Caution:* Do not overload or "lock" your knees.
- **Chest Press (2)** This exercise is also called a bench press. Push upward on the handles, extending your elbows and bring your upper arms toward your chest. This exercise strengthens chest muscles (pectorals) and triceps on the back of your arms. *Note:* Place your feet on the bench with knees and hips flexed and lower back flattened. Do not arch your back.
- **Shoulder Press (3)** This exercise is also called a military press. It strengthens shoulders (deltoids) and backs of your arms (triceps). Push upward on the handles, extending your elbows and bringing your arms toward your ears. *Caution:* Do not arch your back.
- **Lat Pull-Down Bar or High Pulley (4)** To strengthen biceps and latissimus, kneel or stand and pull the bar down behind your neck, alternating with a pull to your chest. To strengthen triceps, perform a "triceps curl" by pulling the bar from chest height to waist or thigh level. Lower your arms, keeping your elbows against your sides.
- **Low Pulley (5)** Perform biceps curls to strengthen your elbow flexor and especially biceps. Stand and pull the handle from thigh level to chest level. Flex your elbows while keeping them close to the sides.
- **Chinning (6)** Chin to strengthen bicep, latissimus, and upper-back muscles. Grasp handles and pull up until your chin is at hand level.
- **Dipping (7)** Dip to strengthen triceps and upper pectorals (chest muscles). Support your weight on the handles, then lower your body by bending your elbows 90°. Push up to a straight-arm position.
- **Abdominal/Tilt Board (9)** Tilt the board at an angle appropriate for your ability. Do bent-knee sit-ups to strengthen upper abdominals.
- **Hamstring Curl (10)** This exercise strengthens your hamstrings and other knee flexors. Lie prone with your heels under the pads. Flex your knees through a full range of motion. You can also do knee extensions by sitting on the end of the bench with ankles under the lower set of pads to strengthen quadriceps and other knee extensors.
- **Back Extension (11)** Use this exercise to strengthen your lower-back muscles. Adjust the apparatus so your feet can be braced while your pelvic bones rest on the pad. Let trunk hang relaxed toward the floor. Extend your back until your trunk is parallel with the floor. *Caution:* Do not arch your back.
- **Low Pulley (12)** Sit with your feet braced, legs straight. Grasp the handles, keeping elbows out at chest level. Pull handles to chest. This strengthens upper back muscles and trapezius. To strengthen lower back muscles, lean trunk backward at your hip joint during the pull.

OTHER STATIONS See your instructor for information on these stations: Hip Flexors (8); Wrist Conditioner (13); Neck Conditioner (14); Hand Gripper (15); Real Runner (16).

8

MUSCULAR ENDURANCE

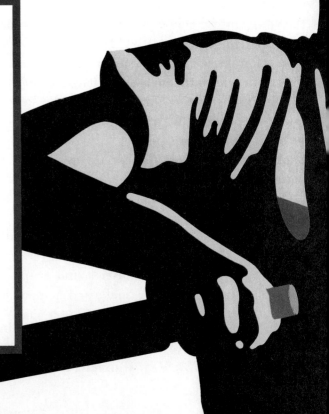

CHAPTER OBJECTIVES

After reading this chapter, you should be able to:

✔ Differentiate among the three types of muscle fibers with regard to function.

✔ Tell how muscular endurance contributes to fitness and good health.

✔ Compare and contrast muscular endurance to other parts of fitness.

✔ Apply the FIT Formula to muscular endurance.

✔ Describe exercises that build muscular endurance.

You already know good cardiovascular fitness can "keep you going" in certain sports and activities. Even when your cardiovascular system is fit, though, you can still tire soon after beginning an activity if you lack muscular endurance. *Muscular endurance* is the ability of the muscles to work for long periods of time without getting tired. In this chapter, you will learn the importance of muscular endurance in sports and everyday life and how to improve your own muscular endurance.

YOUR BODY AND MUSCULAR ENDURANCE

The endurance of a given muscle depends on the kinds of muscle fibers that make up that muscle. Two main kinds of fibers that vary in appearance and function make up all skeletal muscles.

Slow-twitch muscle fibers contract at a slow rate. These fibers contain many structures that release energy. The energy in these fibers is released "aerobically," using oxygen from the blood. Muscles composed mainly of slow-twitch fibers do not tire very easily. They have the greatest endurance of all muscles.

Fast-twitch fibers contract at a fast rate. However, these fibers have fewer energy-releasing structures. Energy is released in these fibers by anaerobic processes—ones that do not use oxygen. Anaerobic processes are less efficient than aerobic ones. So, while muscles composed mainly of fast-twitch fibers have great strength, they are less likely to have endurance.

A third group of fibers, called *intermediate fibers*, have characteristics of both slow- and fast-twitch fibers. They contract at a fast rate and contain many energy-releasing structures. Energy in intermediate fibers is also released aerobically so they, too, have much endurance. But because intermediate fibers contract at a faster rate, muscles containing many intermediate fibers have strength as well as endurance.

The relative number of slow-twitch, fast-twitch, and intermediate fibers in a given muscle is related to that muscle's usual job. The total number of fibers in a muscle does not change, but the kind of exercise you do influences the size of the fibers and their ability to use oxygen. For example, weight training increases size of muscle fibers while bicycling increases their ability to use oxygen.

MUSCULAR ENDURANCE AND FITNESS

People sometimes confuse cardiovascular fitness with muscular endurance. Cardiovascular fitness allows the heart muscle, lungs, and blood vessels to work longer and more efficiently. This results in an improved blood/oxygen delivery system. Muscular endurance allows the skeletal muscles to work longer and more efficiently. This enables you to carry out activities without tiring. Exercising to build cardiovascular fitness helps build some muscular endurance. Cardiovascular exercises improve blood flow to the muscle fibers, which, in turn, aids the muscles' resistance to fatigue and builds their endurance.

Some people think that if you are strong, you automatically have good muscular endurance. While good muscular endurance requires at least some strength, they are not the same. Strength allows the muscles to lift. Endurance allows the muscles to lift for longer periods of time. Strength exercises increase the sizes of muscle fibers, especially the fast-twitch muscle fibers. As the fibers increase in size, the whole muscle increases in size and becomes stronger. Muscular endurance exercises add little to the size of muscle fibers. The ability of muscles to resist fatigue improves because the ability of all fibers to use oxygen improves. With training, even fast-twitch fibers use some oxygen to release energy. As ability to use oxygen improves, muscles use fuel more efficiently and can work for longer periods of time.

You need good muscular endurance to lift light loads repeatedly and to lift or move your own body weight for long periods of time. For example, barbers, dentists, and store clerks stand most of the day. Performing exercises with muscles such as those in the back and neck will help these people avoid getting tired. Similarly, active people such as athletes might exercise muscles in the arms and legs.

Muscular endurance is very important to your everyday life. People with good muscular endurance find it easier to maintain good posture and are less apt to have backaches, muscle soreness, and injuries. Muscular endurance also contributes to good mental health. If you have good muscular endurance, you do not tire easily.

These illustrations show how cardiovascular fitness and muscle strength and endurance benefit you in everyday activities. Having good fitness in all three areas enables you to meet the demands of your job, emergencies, and travel. Notice how you rely on your fitness in one area with each activity. For example, cardiovascular fitness is most important if you must run for help. Muscular strength is needed to move a refrigerator or stove. Muscular endurance enables you to carry a suitcase a long distance without tiring.

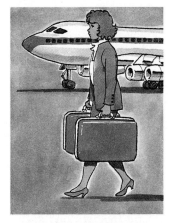

Muscular endurance

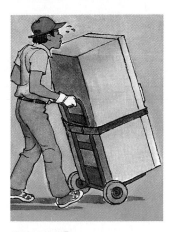

Strength

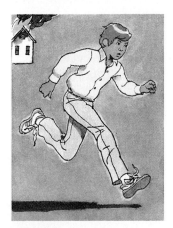

Cardiovascular fitness

THE FIT FORMULA AND MUSCULAR ENDURANCE

The key to achieving muscular endurance is using your muscles for a longer period of time than you normally use them. As you read about each level of muscular endurance, refer to the FIT Formula chart.

Low-intensity exercises can build the muscular endurance needed for daily activities. Exercises at this level give you the endurance to paint a room or shovel snow from a driveway. For this type of endurance, you lift only the body parts you move daily. Examples include raising and lowering your arms, jogging in place, and lifting and lowering your legs while lying on your side. Low intensity is the beginning level when exercising to improve muscular endurance. If you do low-intensity exercises long enough, you might raise your heart rate enough to build cardiovascular fitness as well as muscular endurance.

Medium-intensity exercises can build the muscular endurance needed for good fitness. While low-intensity exercises are a good way to begin developing muscular endurance, many people want to build more muscular endurance. They choose medium-intensity exercises, including body-weight calisthenics such as pull-ups, sit-ups, and knee dips. Medium-intensity exercise allows people to do vigorous activities without tiring quickly and builds some muscle strength. It also helps them maintain a healthy back and good posture. Low- and medium-intensity muscular endurance exercises are all that most people need.

High-intensity exercises can build muscular endurance needed for high-level performance. People who want high-level physical performance usually rely on high-intensity exercise. They choose exercises that increase strength, such as weight training. They can use these exercises to build endurance by increasing the number of repetitions they do, rather than increasing the amount of weight they use.

HAVE YOU HEARD?

Males tend to have more fast-twitch white fibers, while females tend to have more intermediate types. Experts suggest that, with improved training, females will be able to swim and run distances of thirty miles or more with more ease than males.

Fitness Target Zones for Muscular Endurance

	Low Intensity	Medium Intensity	High Intensity
Frequency	Exercise at least 3 days a week; exercise every day for best results.	Exercise at least 3 days a week; exercise every day for best results.	Exercise 3 days a week or every other day.
Intensity	Lift only your own body parts, such as arms and legs.	Lift own body weight.	Lift 20%–70% of the maximum weight you can lift.
Time	Complete at least 9 repetitions over at least 1 minute.	Complete at least 9 repetitions. Increase repetitions gradually to 25. Begin with one set, work up to three sets for advanced muscular endurance.	Complete at least 9 repetitions. Gradually increase from 1 set to 5 sets of 9 to 25 repetitions.

SELF-EVALUATION

MUSCULAR ENDURANCE

WORKSHEET 8-1

Use worksheet 8-1 to record your results of this self-evaluation.

Many exercises can help you evaluate your muscular endurance, but the best ones test your body's large muscles. Follow these directions to evaluate your muscular endurance.

1. Do each of the exercises described below.

2. Record on your worksheet the number of times you completed each exercise. Write *yes* if you could do the exercise as long or as many times as indicated. Write *no* if you could not. If you cannot pass all 5 tests, you need to work on muscular endurance.

3. Look up your rating on the rating chart and record your rating in the space on your worksheet.

Rating Chart: Muscular Endurance

Fitness Rating	Number of tests passed
Good	5
Marginal	3 or 4
Low	less than 3

SIDE STAND

● This exercise tests leg and arm muscles.

1. Lie on your side.

2. Use both hands to get your body supported over your right hand. Keep your body stiff and supported on your right hand and right foot.

3. Raise your left arm and left leg in the air. Males should hold this position for 30 seconds to pass. Females should hold this position for 20 seconds to pass. Return to starting position.

4. Repeat, supporting your body on your left side.

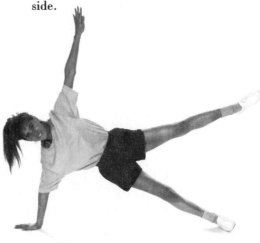

SITTING TUCK

• This exercise tests leg and abdominal muscles.
1. Sit on the floor with your knees bent and arms outstretched.
2. Lean back and balance on your hips. Keep your knees bent near your chest and your feet off the floor.
3. Straighten your knees so your body forms a "V." You can move your arms sideward for balance.
4. Bend your knees to your chest again. Continue pulling your legs in and pushing them out. Count each time you push your legs out. Males should complete 25 repetitions to pass. Females should complete 20 repetitions to pass.

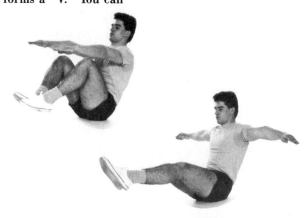

LEG CHANGE

• This exercise tests hip and leg muscles.
1. Get in a push-up position with your weight supported on your hands and feet.
2. Draw your right knee up under your chest, and keep your left leg back.
3. Change legs by pulling your left leg forward and moving your right leg back.
4. Continue changing the legs. *Caution:* Do not let your lower back sag when changing legs. Count each time your right leg comes forward.
5. Repeat this exercise for 1 minute. Both males and females should complete 30 changes with each leg in that time to pass.

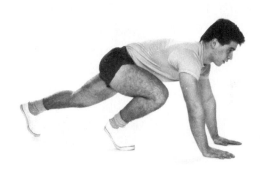

PRONE TRUNK LIFT

• This exercise tests upper back muscles.
1. Lie face down on the floor. Clasp your hands behind your neck. Have a partner hold your feet down with both hands.
2. Lift your head and chest off the floor. *Caution:* Lift slowly. Males should hold this position for 30 seconds to pass. Females should hold this position for 20 seconds to pass. Then return to starting position. *Note:* As a general rule, most people should avoid back-arching exercises. However, there is no harm in arching the back and holding one time as part of a test if you do not have back problems.

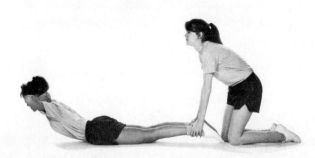

BENT ARM HANG

• This exercise tests arm muscles and shoulder muscles.
1. Hang from a chinning bar. Your palms face away from your body.
2. With the help of a partner, lift your body so your chin is above bar level. Keep your chest close to the bar.
3. Your partner should let go as soon as your chin is above the bar.
4. Males should hold this position for a count of 16 to pass. Females should hold this position for a count of 12 to pass. Begin counting as soon as your partner releases the feet. Stop counting when your chin touches the bar, your head tilts backward, or your chin falls below bar level.

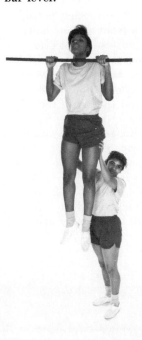

IMPROVING MUSCULAR ENDURANCE

Examples of low- and medium-intensity exercises are shown here. Keep these guidelines in mind before trying these exercises. They can help you avoid soreness or injuries caused by exercising.

● **Begin gradually.** Too much exercise too soon can cause sore muscles. It takes several weeks for your muscles to get accustomed to exercising if they have not been used much. For low-intensity exercises, start below your threshold and gradually work up to your target zone. For medium intensity, start with 9 repetitions and gradually increase the number. If you are sore the next day, repeat some of the same exercises, but complete fewer repetitions.

● **Do not overdo.** Experts feel that there is limited benefit in doing more than 25 repetitions in 1 set. If you are in training for a sport or job and want to do more than 25 repetitions, do them in sets of 25 and rest between sets. Two sets of 25 repetitions each is better than 50 repetitions done in one set. If you want to increase the intensity after 25 repetitions, increase the weight while decreasing repetitions.

● **Do all exercises slowly.** Fast movements can cause joint or muscle injury. You are also more likely to do the exercise incorrectly.

● **Move through a full range of motion.** Moving your muscles and joints through a full range of motion will help keep you more flexible.

STRIDE JUMP

● This low-intensity exercise improves leg muscle and arm muscle endurance.
1. Stand with your right leg forward and left leg back. Hold your left arm nearly straight in front of your body and your right arm nearly straight behind.
2. Jump up, moving your left foot forward and your right foot backward. As your feet change places, your arms should also change position. Whichever arm is forward, the opposite foot should be forward. Keep your feet at least 18 to 24 inches apart.

3. Continue to jump, alternating feet and arms forward and backward. Count 1 each time the right leg comes forward. Try to do 1 jump every 1 to 2 seconds.

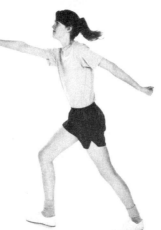

SIDE LEG RAISE

● This low-intensity exercise improves hip muscle and thigh muscle endurance.
1. Lie on your right side. Use your arms to help keep you balanced.
2. Lift your left leg straight up from your side to a 45° angle.

Note: Keep your body and leg straight and stay on your side with your toes facing forward.
3. Lower your leg, and continue repeating the movement.
4. Roll over, and repeat with your right leg.

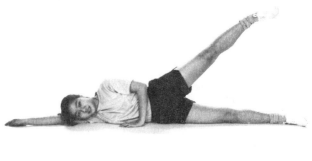

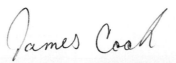

LEG CHANGE

- This low-intensity exercise improves leg, arm, and shoulder muscle endurance. See page 97 for directions. Count 1 each time your right foot comes forward. Try to do 1 leg change every 1 to 2 seconds.

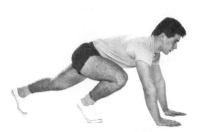

PRONE TRUNK LIFT

- This medium-intensity exercise improves trunk muscle endurance. See page 97 for directions. Try to complete 1 repetition every 1 to 2 seconds. *Caution:* Do not allow the lower end of your sternum to leave the floor.

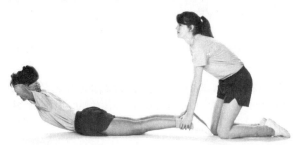

HALF PUSH-UP

- This medium-intensity exercise improves arm and chest muscular endurance. Perform 9 to 25 repetitions. Try to complete 1 repetition every 1 to 4 seconds. If you cannot perform 9, substitute the bent-knee push-up. If you can do more than 25, substitute the push-up (see page 84).

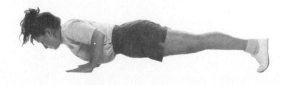

KNEE DIP

- This medium-intensity exercise improves leg muscle endurance. See page 160 for directions. Complete at least 9 repetitions with each leg. Pick a different type of knee dip for muscular endurance than you picked for strength. If you can complete 25 repetitions, try a more difficult knee dip. Try to complete 1 knee dip on each side every 1 to 4 seconds.

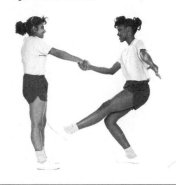

HIGH KNEE JOG IN PLACE

- This medium-intensity exercise improves leg muscle and hip muscle endurance.
1. Jog in one spot. As you jog, try to lift your knees so that your upper leg is lifted parallel to the ground.
2. Count 1 each time your right foot touches the floor. Try to do 1 to 2 jog steps per second.

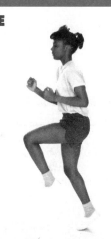

TRUNK CURL (ARMS EXTENDED)

- This medium-intensity exercise develops abdominal muscle endurance. See page 51 for directions. Complete at least 9 repetitions. You will probably have to pick a different form of curl for muscular endurance than you picked for strength. If you can complete 25 curls, choose a more difficult one. Try to complete 1 trunk curl every 1 to 4 seconds.

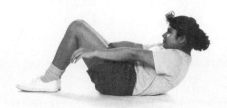

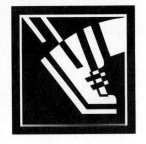

ACTIVITY

MUSCULAR ENDURANCE

Probably no one will ever do all of the muscular-endurance exercises at once. However, everyone should do some muscular-endurance exercises. Use this activity to try several of these exercises so you will have some experience with them. Keep these guidelines in mind:

● Learn how to do each exercise properly.

● Do the exercises in the order and number listed below.

● If you cannot complete an exercise as many times as directed, just do as many as you can. When you design your own program, you can pick the exercise that is best for you.

● Your instructor will tell you when to start the exercise. Between exercises, walk or jog in place to keep active if you finish before others in your group.

● Record on your worksheet each exercise you performed 10 times or for 1 full minute. Record the number you completed or length of time it took you to complete them.

WORKSHEET 8-2

Use worksheet 8-2 to record your results of this activity.

Muscular Endurance Exercises

Exercise	Length of Time or Number of Repetitions
Warm-Up Exercises	Use the warm-up in Chapter 1
Stride Jump	1 every 2 seconds for 1 minute
Side Leg Raise (right leg)	1 every 3 seconds for 1 minute
Side Leg Raise (left leg)	1 every 2 seconds for 1 minute
Leg Change	1 every 3 seconds for 1 minute
Trunk Lift	1 every 2 seconds
Push-Up or Modified Push-Up	10
Knee Dip	1 every 2 seconds for 1 minute
High Knee Jog in Place	10
Lower Knee Jog	1 every 2 seconds for 1 minute
Trunk Curl (Arms Extended)	20
Walk in a Circle	2 minutes

CHAPTER REVIEW

MULTIPLE CHOICE
Choose the letter of the best answer.

1. If you become tired, but not winded, after vigorous exercise, you might lack good (a) muscular endurance. (b) body fatness. (c) flexibility. (d) cardiovascular fitness.

2. Exercises that develop fast-twitch muscle fibers seem to affect a muscle's (a) strength. (b) reaction time. (c) endurance. (d) flexibility.

3. Which is a medium-intensity exercise? (a) weight lifting (b) jogging in place (c) side leg raise (d) half pull-up

4. Which is probably the most important factor related to muscular endurance? (a) heart rate (b) blood flow rate (c) muscle size (d) type of muscle fibers

5. Which probably requires strength more than it does muscular endurance? (a) jogging (b) tennis (c) hiking (d) weight lifting

6. Which best describes how strength and muscular endurance are related? (a) opposite (b) similar (c) identical (d) not closely related

7. How can exercise benefit muscle fibers? (a) decreases size of muscle fibers (b) increases efficiency of oxygen use (c) increases number of muscle fibers (d) makes muscles thinner

8. At which level should a beginner start doing low-intensity exercises? (a) below threshold of training (b) at threshold of training (c) at target zone (d) above target zone

9. When exercising for endurance, what is the minimum number of repetitions that should be done in one set? (a) 5 (b) 9 (c) 15 (d) 25

10. Which helps develop low-intensity muscular endurance? (a) trunk lift (b) pull-up (c) jog in place (d) knee dip

MATCHING
Match the definition in Column I with the term it defines in Column II.

Column I
11. fibers in a muscle likely to have muscular endurance
12. needed for good fitness
13. needed for high-level performance
14. needed for daily activities
15. ability to lift for longer periods of time

Column II
a. high-intensity exercises
b. low-intensity exercises
c. medium-intensity exercises
d. muscular endurance
e. slow-twitch muscle fiber

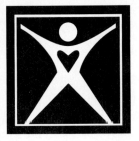

FOCUS ON FITNESS

HOMEMADE WEIGHTS

Weight training is an excellent way to build strength and muscular endurance. However, weight-training equipment is usually quite expensive. If your goal is to build moderate levels of strength and muscular endurance, you can make your own weights. You will need these materials:

● a strong broomstick or dowel rod at least 3/4 of an inch to 1 inch in diameter and 5 to 7 feet long

● 6 plastic milk or bleach bottles with caps and open handles

Partially fill each bottle with water or sand. Weigh each bottle on a bathroom scale. You might use these amounts: 2 bottles with about 2 pounds of water or sandeach; 2 bottles with about 4 pounds of water or sand each; 2 bottles with about 5 pounds of water or sand each. Use a felt-tip marker to write the weight on each bottle. You can lift the bottles through their handles or slip the broomstick through the bottles' handles to make a barbell.

Caution: Do not use homemade barbells for heavy lifting; the broomstick could break or the weights could slip off the ends of the broomstick. Do not lift more than 15 pounds at a time. Do not put more bottles on the broomstick than can slide on easily, yet still be manageable. Finally, remember to warm up before exercising and to cool down after exercising.

BICEPS CURL

1. Hold the stick with your palms up.
2. Lift your arms up to your shoulders. Keep your elbows in to your sides.
3. Lower your arms.
4. Return to starting position. Repeat 3 to 15 times. Complete 1 to 3 sets.

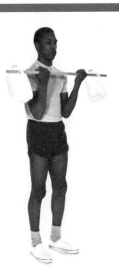

TOE RAISE

1. Stand with the balls of your feet on a board about 2 inches high. Keep your feet positioned so your toes are turned in slightly. Rest the stick and weights on your shoulders.
2. Press with your feet until your heels lift off the floor.
3. Return to starting position. Repeat 3 to 15 times. Complete 1 to 3 sets.

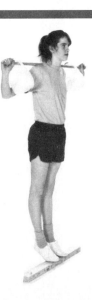

ARM RAISE

1. Hold the stick and weights in your hands.
2. Lift your arms and hands above your head.
3. Return to starting position. Repeat 3 to 15 times. Complete 1 to 3 sets.

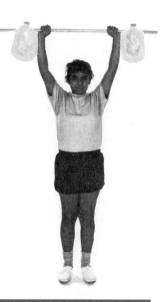

MILITARY PRESS

1. Hold the stick and weights at shoulder height with the palms of your hands facing away.
2. Push your arms above your head.
3. Return to starting position. Repeat 3 to 15 times. Complete 1 to 3 sets.

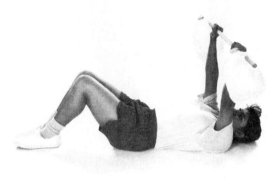

HALF-SQUAT

1. Stand with the stick and weights resting on your shoulders.
2. Squat so that your upper legs are parallel to the floor. *Caution:* Do not squat lower than parallel to the floor.
3. Return to starting position. Repeat 3 to 15 times. Complete 1 to 3 sets.

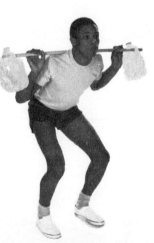

SHOULDER SHRUG

1. Hold the stick and weights with your arms hanging to your sides, palms facing your body.
2. Lift your shoulders and slowly roll them backward.
3. Slowly return to starting position. Repeat 3 to 15 times. Complete 1 to 3 sets.

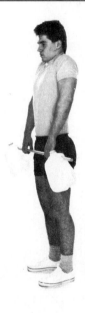

9

FLEXIBILITY

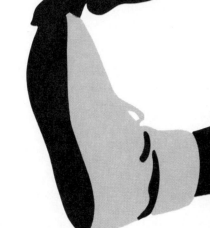

CHAPTER OBJECTIVES

After reading this chapter, you should be able to:

✔ Explain the importance of good flexibility.

✔ Describe safe, effective stretching exercises.

✔ Apply the parts of the FIT Formula to flexibility.

✔ List cautions when stretching.

If you have watched track-and-field events, you noticed that the athletes stretch and "warm up." They make sure that their joints and muscles can move freely before competing.

At various places in your body, bones come together to form *joints*. Your ankles, knees, hips, wrists, elbows, and shoulders are examples of joints. Some joints work like hinges, permitting movement in only two directions. Other joints work like a ball and socket, allowing movement in all directions. Some joints allow a wide range of motion; others allow only limited motion.

Flexibility is the ability to move your joints through a full range of movement. Good flexibility helps you perform activities more easily than does poor flexibility. It also reduces your risk of soreness or muscle injury. If you do not maintain flexibility, your muscles become shorter or "tighter," and movement becomes limited. In this chapter, you will learn more about the importance of good flexibility and how to evaluate and improve your own flexibility.

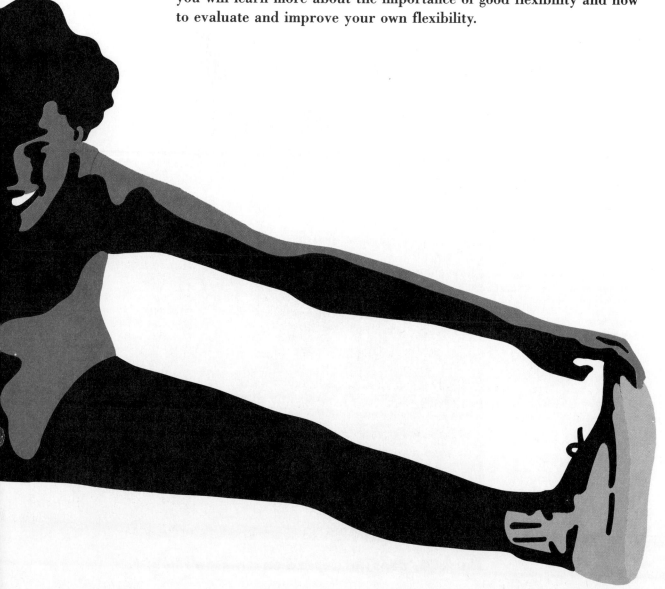

FLEXIBILITY AND GOOD HEALTH

Everyone needs a minimum amount of flexibility to maintain good health and mobility. Some people need additional flexibility because their daily activities require it. For example, cheerleaders, dancers, and gymnasts need to be flexible to perform their routines. Plumbers, painters, carpenters, and mechanics often need to bend and stretch to reach out-of-the-way places.

PHYSICAL BUILD AND FLEXIBILITY Some people mistakenly think that shorter persons can touch their toes more easily than taller persons. A shorter person tends to have relatively short legs and a short trunk, but the person also tends to have shorter arms. In contrast, a tall person tends to have longer legs and trunk, as well as longer arms. Studies have shown that females tend to be more flexible than males. Young people tend to be more flexible than older people.

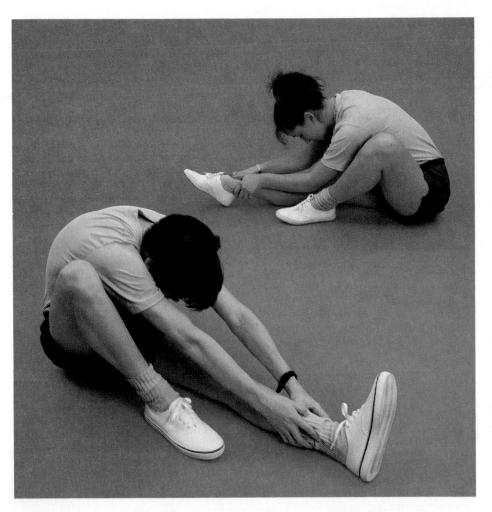

Flexibility does not depend on a person's height.

STRENGTH AND FLEXIBILITY Strength and flexibility can complement each other. By performing flexibility exercises while also working to improve strength, you can avoid becoming muscle-bound—a condition in which one or more joints are limited in their range of motion by muscles that are too short. On the other hand, if you exercise just for flexibility and do not maintain muscle strength, you increase your risk of injury. For example, consider the knee joint. It is surrounded by muscles and *ligaments*—tough, white tissue that connects bones. Your knee is designed to bend in only one direction. If the muscles and ligaments around this joint are stretched too far, the joint becomes "loose" and the knee joint could dislocate. Strong muscles around the knee can help prevent such injuries.

An exercise program should include activities to strengthen all your muscle groups, so your muscles pull with equal force in all directions. For example, if you always strengthen your pectoral muscles on the front of your chest and never strengthen your upper back muscles, you could lose flexibility in your shoulder joints. Your pectoral muscles will pull your shoulders forward. The result is poor posture. At the same time, your pectoral muscles will become "tight"; you will be unable to easily pull your shoulders back.

FITNESS PRINCIPLES AND FLEXIBILITY

You can apply the principles of overload, progression, and specificity (discussed in Chapter 4) as you exercise to improve your flexibility. Each principle plays an important role in increasing flexibility.

PRINCIPLE OF OVERLOAD You must stretch your muscles farther than you normally stretch them to increase your flexibility. Certain stretching exercises make use of gravity or your own body weight to increase flexibility. For example, when you bend over to touch your toes, the weight of your upper body helps you reach farther than you would if you were sitting and tried to touch your toes. You could also sit and hold your ankles, and use your arms to pull yourself forward and stretch your legs. A partner could also help you stretch your muscles, though this action must be carefully and correctly performed.

PRINCIPLE OF PROGRESSION Like other parts of fitness, you must gradually make each flexibility exercise more difficult. Start with a few easy stretches, and gradually stretch farther and longer each day. Doing so will help you prevent muscle soreness and injury.

PRINCIPLE OF SPECIFICITY Flexibility exercises improve only the specific muscles and joints that you stretch. To develop overall flexibility, you must stretch all of your body's muscles, and use all of your body's joints regularly.

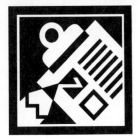

SELF-EVALUATION

FLEXIBILITY

WORKSHEET 9-1

Use worksheet 9-1 to record and interpret your results.

Use this self-evaluation to help you evaluate the flexibility of muscles and joints that you are most likely to use. The sit-and-reach measures the flexibility of your back muscles and the muscles that cross the back of your hip and knee. Use the arm lift to measure the flexibility of muscles on the front of your shoulder joints. The prone trunk lift measures the flexibility of muscles in your upper back and trunk. Use the rating chart to evaluate your flexibility. Once you have evaluated your flexibility, exercise to maintain or increase it. Follow these guidelines when evaluating your flexibility:

● Perform each test shown here.

● Record your score on your worksheet. Use only the "First Trial" part of your worksheet. You are expected to do these tests in class only once unless your instructor tells you otherwise. However, retest yourself periodically. Your worksheet provides space to record additional results when you retest yourself in the future.

Rating Chart: Flexibility

Fitness Rating	Sit and Reach	Arm Lift	Prone Trunk Lift
High Performance	13 or more	14 or more	18 or more
Good	10–12	11–13	14–17
Marginal	8–9	8–10	10–13
Low	7 or less	7 or less	9 or less

BACK-SAVER SIT AND REACH

1. Place a yardstick on top of a 12 inch high box. Have the yardstick extend 9 inches over the box toward you.
2. Sit with your feet against the box.
3. Keep your right leg straight. Bend your left knee until your left foot is flat on the floor. Make sure your left knee is on the outside of your left arm. Your left knee may rotate outward to allow you to reach forward.
4. Reach as far as you can. Hold your reach for 3 seconds. Have a partner read on the yardstick the distance you reach. This number is your score. For example, if you can reach your toes and hold your reach for 3 seconds, your score is 9.
5. Repeat with each leg.
6. Record your score.

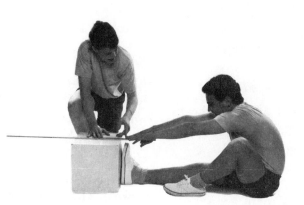

PRONE TRUNK LIFT

Note: Do this part in groups of 3.
1. Lie face down with your legs together. Have one partner hold your feet down. Clasp your hands behind your neck.
2. Lift your chin and chest as high as possible. Hold the position for 3 seconds.
3. Have the second partner use a yardstick to measure the distance from the floor to your chin.
4. Record your score on your worksheet.

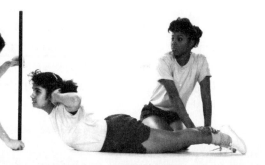

ARM LIFT

1. Lie face down on the floor. Hold a broomstick or other stick above your head at shoulder width. Keep your palms down and arms and wrists straight.
2. Raise your arms and the stick as high as possible. Keep your chin on the floor and your wrists straight during the lift. Use a tight fist to hold the stick.
3. Hold the position for 3 seconds. Have your partner use a yardstick to measure the distance from the floor to the bottom of the stick, as shown here. Your score is this distance.
4. Record your score on your worksheet.

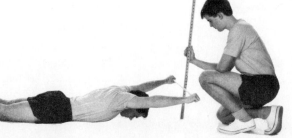

ACHIEVING BETTER FLEXIBILITY

Stretching correctly and safely is one of the best ways to improve your flexibility. You may want to include both static stretching and ballistic stretching in your exercise program.

STATIC STRETCHING *Static stretching* is stretching slowly as far as you can without pain, and then holding the stretch for several seconds. Done correctly, static stretching increases your flexibility and can help you relax. Static stretching exercises are safer than ballistic exercises since you are less likely to stretch too far and injure yourself. Static stretching can be especially beneficial to people who have bad backs, previous muscle or joint injuries, or arthritis. Even athletes should perform static stretches at the beginning and end of their exercise programs to warm up and cool down. By themselves, static stretches might not build enough flexibility for an athlete, so ballistic stretches might be needed.

BALLISTIC STRETCHING *Ballistic stretching* is a series of quick but gentle bouncing or bobbing-type motions that are *not* held for a long time. If you are active in sports, it is important that part of your exercise program include movements that are used in your sports. If you move or stretch muscles quickly in a sport (for example, fast throwing or sprinting), then some of your flexibility exercises should resemble the sport's movement. While ballistic stretching might be more effective than static stretching, you must be careful to stretch gently. Stretching too quickly or overstretching can cause injury. This chart shows the flexibility benefits of many sports and other activities.

HAVE YOU HEARD?

Note that many of the sports listed in the chart are rated "poor" for building flexibility. In most sports, it is the training for the sport, not the sport itself, that develops flexibility in the participants.

Flexibility Benefits

Sport or Activity	Benefit	Sport or Activity	Benefit	Sport or Activity	Benefit
Aerobics	good	Fencing	fair	Sailing	poor
Aqua Dynamics	fair	Football	poor	Skating; Ice or Roller	poor
Archery	poor	Golf (walking)	fair	Skiing	
Backpacking	fair	Gymnastics	excellent	Cross-Country	poor
Badminton	fair	Hiking	fair	Downhill	poor
Baseball	poor	Horseback Riding	poor	Soccer	fair
Basketball (half court)	poor	Interval Training	poor	Softball (fast pitch)	poor
(vigorous)	poor	Jogging	poor	(slow pitch)	poor
Bowling	poor	Judo/Karate	fair	Surfing	fair
Canoeing	poor	Mountain Climbing	poor	Swimming	fair
Circuit Training	good	Pool/Billiards	poor	Table Tennis	poor
Continuous Rhythmical		Racquetball/Handball	poor	Tennis	poor
Exercise	good	Rope Jumping	poor	Volleyball	poor
Dance		Rowing; crew	poor	Walking	poor
Aerobic	good			Waterskiing	poor
Ballet	excellent			Weight Training	poor
Modern	excellent				
Social	poor				

THE FIT FORMULA AND FLEXIBILITY

To improve the flexibility of your joints and increase the length of your muscles, you must exercise in the fitness target zone for flexibility. Flexibility has two different target zones: one for static exercise and one for ballistic exercise.

Fitness Target Zones for Flexibility

	Static	Ballistic
Frequency	• Stretch each muscle groups daily, if possible, but at least 3 days a week. Stretch before and after workouts.	• Stretch each muscle group daily, if possible, but at least 3 days a week if you are an athlete.
Intensity	• The muscle must be stretched beyond its normal length. • You must have a partner or equipment, or you can use your own body weight to assist you to have an overload.	• The muscle must be stretched beyond its normal length. • Use slow, *gentle* bounces or bobs, using the motion of your body part to stretch the specific muscle. *Caution:* No stretch should cause pain, especially sharp pain. Be especially careful when doing ballistic stretching.
Time	• Hold each stretch for 10 to 15 seconds. • Stretch each muscle group for 3 sets of 10 to 15 seconds each.	• Bounce against the muscle slowly and *gently* 6 to 12 times. • Stretch each muscle group for 3 sets of 6 to 12 repetitions each.

EXERCISING TO IMPROVE FLEXIBILITY

Jogging, swimming, tennis, and other activities or sports do much to improve your cardiovascular fitness, strength, and muscle endurance. However, you must perform specific exercises to improve your flexibility. Some flexibility exercises can help relieve muscle soreness. A *muscle cramp*—the sudden spasm, or tightening, of a muscle—can make a muscle sore. Slow stretching can help relieve this tightness.

The exercises below can help improve your flexibility in all parts of your body. Note that the exercises can be performed either statically or ballistically. However, before you begin stretching, keep these cautions and guidelines in mind:

● Experts suggest you do mild exercise, such as walking or slow jogging, to warm up before stretching.

● Start with static stretching if you do not exercise regularly or did not get a high performance rating on the self-evaluation.

● Do *not* stretch ballistically if you have a previous injury or back problem. Use static stretches only.

● Do *not* stretch until you feel pain. Stretch only until the muscle feels "tight" and a little uncomfortable, but *not* painful.

● To benefit from static stretching, you usually need a weight or some outside force, such as a partner, to provide an overload. If you use partners, they should be *extremely careful* not to overstretch you.

● When possible, use your own muscles to stretch another muscle. For example, contract the muscles on the front of your thighs to help pull and stretch muscles in the backs of your legs.

● If you are an athlete performing ballistic stretches, do *not* get over-enthusiastic and try to bounce too far. Stretch gently to avoid injury.

● Start slowly. Even though stretching might seem very easy to do, you should begin slowly and gradually increase the length of time you stretch or the number of times you repeat a stretch.

TRUNK TWISTER

● This exercise stretches your trunk and hip muscles.

Static Stretch
1. Sit with your left leg straight. Bend your right leg and cross it over your left leg. Place your right foot flat on the floor next to your left knee.
2. Place your left arm on the right side of your bent knee and press on it. Place your right hand on the floor behind you.

3. Twist your trunk as far as possible and look over your right shoulder. Hold the position

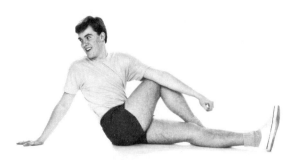

for 10 to 15 seconds.
4. Reverse your arm and leg positions and repeat.

Ballistic Stretch
● Follow the same procedure as for the static stretch, but make these changes:
1. After getting into position, instead of holding, gently bounce 6 times by pushing your right elbow against your left knee and pulling your left shoulder back.
2. Reverse your arm and leg positions and repeat.

ARM REACH

• This exercise stretches your shoulder and chest muscles.

Static Stretch

1. Sit on the floor or on a bench. Keep your chin in and your back straight. Have a partner stand and place his/her knee between your shoulder blades.

2. Raise your arms to shoulder level. Bend your elbows to point back at your partner.
3. After you pull your elbows back as far as possible, have your partner gently pull them back *slightly* farther. Hold the position for 10 to 15 seconds.

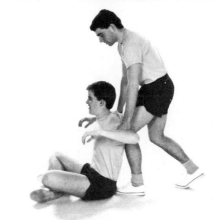

Ballistic Stretch

1. Sit on the floor or on a bench. Keep your chin in and your back straight. Raise your arms to shoulder level and bend your elbows so they point sideways.
2. Touch your fists in front of your chest. Then jerk your elbows backward. Return to starting position.
3. Fling your arms back again, straightening your elbows. Alternate the bent-arm jerk with straight arm fling.
4. Count 1 repetition each time you move your bent elbows back. Complete 6 repetitions. *Caution:* Be sure your head does not go forward when your arms go back.

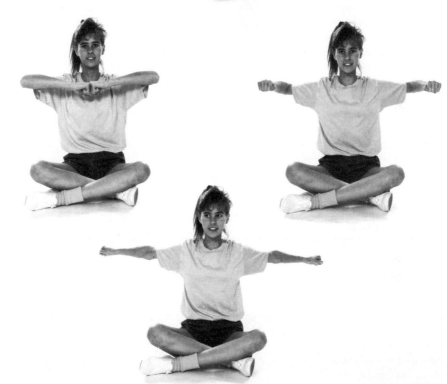

SIDE STRETCHER

• This exercise stretches your trunk muscles.

Static Stretch

1. Stand with your feet about 12 inches apart. Hold your right hand behind your neck. Hold 10 pounds of weight in your left hand, down at your side.
2. Bend as far as you can to your left side. Try to lower the weight to knee level or lower.

Hold the position for 10 to 15 seconds.
3. Hold the weight in your right hand and repeat the stretch on your right side. *Caution:* Do *not* twist your spine or bend forward or backward.

Ballistic Stretch

• Follow the same procedure as for the static

stretch, but make these changes:
1. Do *not* use the weight.
2. Bounce up and down gently after you have reached as far as you can to your left side. Bounce 6 times. Then change sides and repeat on your right side. *Caution:* Do *not* twist your spine or bend forward or backward.

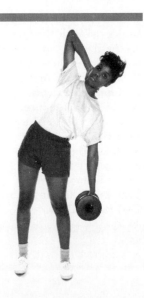

CALF STRETCHER

● This exercise stretches your calf muscles and Achilles tendon.

Static Stretch
Part A
1. Assume a lunge position. Your right knee should be bent and forward. Your left leg should be straight and back as far as possible; your left foot remains flat on the floor, heel down. Rest your hands on your right knee.
2. Hold the position for 10 to 15 seconds. Keep your left knee straight and heel down.
3. Change legs and repeat procedure.

Part B
● Follow the same procedure as for Part A, but make these changes:
1. Bend the knee of your back leg and shift your weight on to it.
2. Keep your foot flat on floor, heel down. You should feel a pull in your Achilles tendon.

Ballistic Stretch
Part A
● Follow the same procedure as for the static stretch, but make these changes:
1. Stretch your left leg backward with the toes on the floor. *Gently* try to force your heel to the floor. Bounce 6 times.
2. Change legs and repeat the procedure.

Part B
● Follow the same procedure as Part A, but gently bounce on your back knee, keeping your heel on the floor.

LOW BACK STRETCHER

● This exercise stretches the muscles of your lower back. It is only done statically.
1. Lie on your back and bring both knees to your chest.
2. Use your arms to squeeze your knees toward your chest. Hold this position for 6 to 15 seconds.

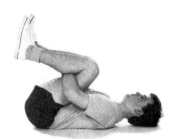

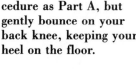

HIP AND THIGH STRETCHER

● This exercise stretches muscles on the front of your hip joint.

Static Stretch

1. Kneel on your left knee. Keep your right knee directly above your right ankle. Stretch your left leg back. Place your hands on the floor.
2. Keep your left knee on the floor as you shift your pelvis and trunk forward. You should feel a pull on the front of your left hip joint. Hold this position for 10 to 15 seconds.
3. Change your leg position and repeat with your right leg.

Ballistic Stretch

● Follow the same procedure as for the static stretch, but make these changes:
1. Gently bounce at your pelvis 6 times.
2. Then change your leg position and bounce 6 times on your right leg.

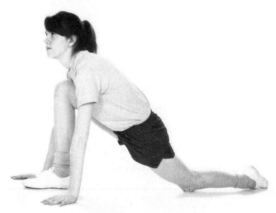

BACK-SAVER TOE TOUCH

● This exercise stretches muscles on the back of your hips and legs. It is a better flexibility exercise than the sit-and-reach test used in the self-evaluation since it places less stretch on your back and more on the leg. The self-evaluation test is safe to use one time as a test, but it is not recommended as an exercise for your workout. This exercise is only done statically, not ballistically.

1. Sit on the floor with your right leg straight. Bend your left leg and place your left foot flat on floor.
2. Grasp your right ankle with both hands. Pull with your arms. Try to touch your head to your knee. Hold the position for 15 seconds.
3. Repeat with your left leg straight and your right knee bent.

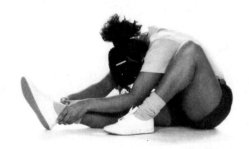

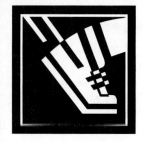

ACTIVITY

FLEXIBILITY

Now that you know the importance of good flexibility, review your results of the self-evaluation on pages 108–109. Then use the flexibility exercises described on pages 112 through 115 to improve your flexibility. If you did not get a "good fitness" or a "high performance" rating on the self-evaluation, or if you have been inactive or have an old injury, choose the static exercises. If you rated "good fitness" or "high performance" and exercise regularly, you should begin with static stretches, but might want to include ballistic stretches as well. Follow these guidelines while completing this activity:

● Record the date you exercise on your worksheet. You will probably perform only one set of each exercise during class, but the worksheet has room to record your results for several weeks.

● Hold the position of each static exercise for 10 to 15 seconds. Complete 6 repetitions of each ballistic exercise.

● Gradually increase each static exercise from 10 to 15 seconds, and increase each ballistic exercise from 6 to 12 bounces during the next 4 to 6 weeks.

● Start with 1 set of each exercise and gradually increase your number of repetitions. When you can hold a static-exercise position for 15 seconds, or complete 12 bounces of a ballistic exercise without making your muscles sore, increase your repetitions to 2 sets. Later, increase your repetititons to 3 sets when you can do so without discomfort.

WORKSHEET 9-2

Use worksheet 9-2 to record your results of this activity.

Flexibility Exercises	
Exercise	**Page**
Trunk Twister	112
Side Stretcher	113
Arm Reach	113
Calf Stretcher	114
Low Back Stretcher	114
Hip and Thigh Stretcher	115
Back-Saver Toe Touch	115

CHAPTER REVIEW

MULTIPLE CHOICE
Choose the letter of the best answer.

1. Flexibility is the (a) ability to exercise for long periods of time without tiring. (b) amount of force you can exert with your muscles. (c) ability to complete many repetitions of an exercise without tiring. (d) ability to move your joints through a full range of motion.

2. The difference between static and ballistic flexibility exercises is the (a) number of times and speed with which exercise is done. (b) specific muscles that are stretched. (c) kind of strength you have. (d) amount of flexibility you need.

3. You can increase a muscle's flexibility by (a) running an extra lap around a track. (b) lifting as heavy a weight as you can. (c) stretching the muscle farther than it is normally stretched. (d) stretching the muscle less than you normally would.

4. Inactive people should begin increasing flexibility with (a) static stretching. (b) ballistic stretching. (c) both static and ballistic stretching. (d) stationary stretching.

5. The FIT Formula for flexibility applies to what kinds of stretching? (a) both static and ballistic (b) static only (c) ballistic only (d) neither static nor ballistic

6. Which exercise helps improve your flexibility? (a) leg raise (b) isometric (c) isotonic (d) trunk twister

7. A good fitness program should include (a) flexibility exercises only. (b) strength exercises only. (c) cardiovascular exercises only. (d) a combination of exercises.

8. Ballistic stretching (a) involves bouncing motion. (b) is safer than static stretching. (c) improves back injuries. (d) should be avoided.

9. Movement is limited when your muscles are (a) longer. (b) shorter. (c) heavier. (d) thinner.

10. Flexibility exercises (a) help you become muscle-bound. (b) increase the flexibility of few muscles and joints. (c) should gradually increase in difficulty. (d) are unimportant to good fitness.

MATCHING
Match the definition in Column I with the term it defines in Column II.

Column I
11. place where two bones meet
12. tough tissue that connects bones
13. stretching slowly without pain
14. stretching that includes bouncing motions
15. sudden tightening of a muscle

Column II
a. ballistic stretching
b. joint
c. ligament
d. muscle cramp
e. static stretching

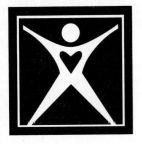

FOCUS ON FITNESS

IMPROVING YOUR FLEXIBILITY

Just as maintaining muscular endurance and cardiovascular fitness are lifelong commitments, so is maintaining and improving your flexibility. You can develop flexibility through calisthenics and sports, but you can also work with a partner to improve flexibility. Most of the activities on these two pages require a partner. Choose a partner who is about your height and weight.

POSTURE STRETCH

● This exercise improves your upper back flexibility.
1. Sit back to back with your partner. Raise both arms overhead. Clasp your partner's hands.
2. Have your partner lean forward *very slowly* and *gently* pull your arms. You should relax and let your head and trunk lean backward. Be sure to tell your partner when to stop pulling.
3. Hold your position for 10 seconds.
4. Take turns repeating this procedure. Each person should complete 3 repetitions.

STICK JUMP

● This exercise improves flexibility in your shoulders, trunk, hips, and legs.
1. Use both hands to hold a length of broomstick or thick dowel rod in front of your thighs. Your hands should be a little farther apart than shoulder width.
2. Jump high and swing the stick under your feet and behind your body without losing your grip.
3. Jump over the stick again, this time swinging the stick back toward the front of your body. *Caution:* This activity is most safely done on a gymnastics mat or other surface that will "give" in case you fall.

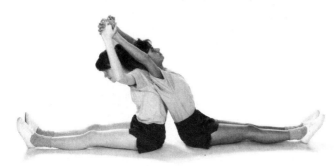

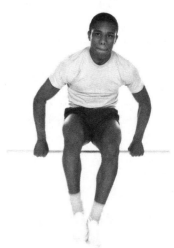

WRING THE DISH TOWEL

● This exercise improves flexibility in your shoulders, hips, and trunk.

1. Stand facing your partner. Hold each other's hands.

2. Start with your left foot while your partner starts with the right foot. Crouch slightly and without releasing hands, take turns stepping over your left arm (partner's right) and into the middle of the "hole" formed by your arms.

3. Turn back to back, swinging your arms overhead without releasing your grip.

4. Continue to turn and then both step out of the "hole" with the other legs. You should finish facing each other and still holding hands.

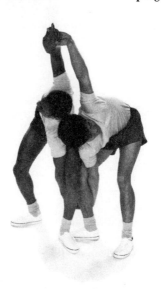 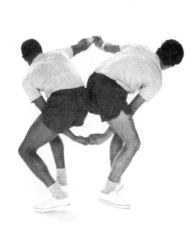 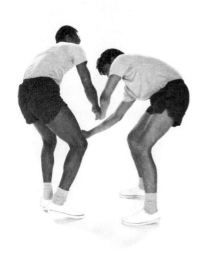

BACK TOUCH

● This exercise improves flexibility in your shoulders.

1. Reach your right hand over your right shoulder and down your spine as if you were pulling up a zipper. Hold this position while you reach your left hand behind your back, bend your elbow and reach up your spine.

2. Clasp your fingers or touch your fingers.

3. Repeat the procedure, this time reaching with your left hand over your left shoulder.

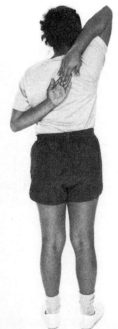

WRAP AROUND

● This exercise improves shoulder and neck flexibility.

1. Reach your right hand behind your head. Try to touch the left corner of your mouth. You can turn your head if needed.

2. Repeat the procedure, using your left hand to touch the right corner of your mouth.

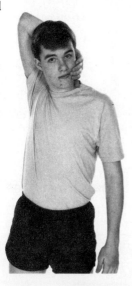

10

EXERCISE AND
FAT CONTROL

CHAPTER OBJECTIVES

After reading this chapter, you should
be able to:

✔ Describe an ideal level of body fat.

✔ Explain how the level of body fat is
related to good health.

✔ Explain how to maintain an ideal
level of body fat.

The human body is made up of many tissues, including muscles, bones, and body organs such as the liver, kidneys, and lungs. Another kind of body tissue is fat. In this chapter you will learn about the importance of body fat, how your level of body fat affects your health, and how to regulate your level of body fat.

ESSENTIAL BODY FAT

The minimum amount of body fat that a person should possess is called *essential body fat.* If fat levels in the body drop below the essential body-fat level, health problems can result.

Your body needs a certain amount of fat. Fat is an insulator, because it helps your body adapt to heat and cold. Fat also acts as a shock absorber that can protect your body organs and bones from injury. Finally, fat is stored energy that is available when your body needs it. Having too little fat can result in abnormal functioning of various body organs. Not only does fat affect health, but most people think having a certain amount of body fat makes you look better.

Having too much fat also can be unhealthful. Scientists tell us that people who have too much body fat have a higher risk of heart disease, high blood pressure, diabetes, and other diseases. An overfat person has less chance of successful surgery, tires more quickly than a leaner person, and might be less efficient in work and recreation.

With respect to fitness, the terms "underweight" and "overweight" do not provide a great deal of information. Underweight and overweight refer to how much you weigh compared to someone else. However, muscles weigh more than fat. Thus, you can weigh more than someone else about the same size because you are more muscular and have less body fat than the other person. Or, you can weigh less than someone else about the same size because you have smaller bones.

On the other hand, the terms "overfat" and "underfat" are very useful because they describe how much of your total body weight is made up of fat. *Underfat* means having too little body fat; *overfat* means having too much body fat. *Obesity* is a term used to describe people who are very overfat.

INFLUENCES ON BODY-FAT LEVELS

Heredity, childhood, and adolescence can play a part in determining the percentage of body fat a person has. While inherited traits cannot be changed, percentages of body fat during childhood and adolescence can be influenced.

HEREDITY Scientists know that people inherit their body type from their parents. This means that they are born with a tendency to be lean, muscular, or fat. For this reason, it is harder for some people to gain weight. Of course, inherited tendencies also make it harder for some people to control body fatness. However, heredity is not nearly as important in determining body type as what you eat and how much you exercise.

EARLY FATNESS Fat children and teenagers are more likely to become fat adults. To prevent being a fat adult, you must do something about overfatness very early in life. Young people who are overfat develop extra fat cells that make it easier to get fat later in life. A person with extra fat cells can lose the fat and keep it off, but it is more difficult for them to do so than it is for other people.

MAINTAINING OPTIMAL BODY FATNESS

The amount you eat and the amount you exercise are the major factors in achieving and maintaining an ideal level of body fat. To many people, the word "diet" means a weight-loss program. In this book, however, *diet* generally refers to a person's eating habits.

DIET When you eat, you take in Calories. The *Calorie*, a heat unit, refers to the energy available in food. A typical male your age needs to consume about 2,500 to 3,000 Calories per day to maintain an ideal level of body fat. A female your age needs about 2,000 to 2,500 Calories per day to maintain an ideal level of body fat. This difference is partly because males are larger in body size and have a greater amount of muscle mass.

EXERCISE When you exercise, your body burns Calories for energy. Every activity uses some Calories. The more vigorous an activity, the more Calories your body burns. When you increase your exercise, you increase the number of Calories you consume for your body to burn, or your body uses stored Calories in fat.

An inactive person uses less energy each day and therefore needs to consume fewer Calories. A very active person, such as a professional soccer player, uses many more Calories per day than an average person. As a result, a very active person needs to consume more Calories than the average person.

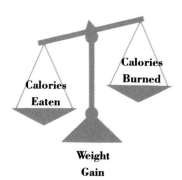

Weight
Gain

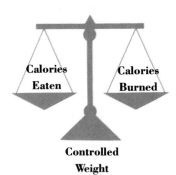

Controlled
Weight

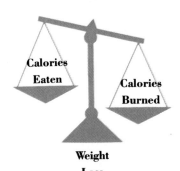

Weight
Loss

Calorie consumption and use

GAINING OR LOSING BODY FAT

Every food you eat contains Calories. Of course, some foods have more Calories than other foods. The more Calories a food has, the more fattening it is. Since fat is stored energy (stored Calories), one way to lose fat is to take in fewer Calories than your body needs or uses. A pound of fat contains 3,500 Calories. Therefore, you can lose a pound of fat by eating 3,500 Calories less than you normally do in a given time. You can also gain a pound of fat by eating 3,500 Calories more than you usually eat in a given time.

Exercise can help control your level of body fat. Since your body works harder than normal when you exercise, it uses additional Calories during exercise. People who feel they are too thin, but do not have eating disorders (such as anorexia nervosa or bulimia), can gain weight by consuming additional Calories. Exercise, particularly strength-building exercise, can also benefit these individuals by helping build muscle. Eating more and doing this kind of exercise can help increase weight and make a person look his or her best without causing unnecessary gains in body fat. For those people who inherited lean body types, it will take a while to "fill out," but the combination of proper diet, proper exercise, and physical development during adolescence will do the job.

THE FIT FORMULA AND FAT CONTROL

Both diet and exercise play an important role in maintaining an ideal level of body fat. Because diet and exercise are important in fat control, each has a fitness target zone as shown below.

Fitness Target Zones for Fat Control

	Diet	Exercise
Frequency	• Eat 3 regular meals daily or 4 or 5 small meals. Regular, controlled eating is best for losing fat. Skipping meals and snacking is usually not effective.	• Exercise daily. Regular exercise is best for losing fat. Short or irregular exercise does little for controlling body fat.
Intensity	• To lose a pound of fat, you must eat 3,500 calories less than normal. • To gain a pound of fat, you must eat 3,500 Calories more than normal. • To maintain your weight, you must keep the number of Calories you eat the same.	• To lose a pound of fat, you must use 3,500 Calories more than normal. • To gain a pound of fat, you must use 3,500 Calories less than normal. • To maintain your weight, you must keep your exercise level.
Time	Neither diet nor exercise results in quick fat loss. Medical specialists recommend that a person lose no more than 1 or 2 pounds of weight per week without medical supervision. Both diet and exercise can be used to safely lose 1 or 2 pounds per week.	

WHAT IS AN IDEAL LEVEL OF BODY FAT?

About one-half of your body fat is located deep within your body. The remaining fat is between your skin and muscles. A fit person has an ideal amount of body fat—neither too much nor too little.

From the late teens on, females generally have a higher percentage of body fat than do males. For females, less than 11 percent is considered too little body fat. Scientists think that having less than this amount of body fat can contribute to problems in a female's reproductive system. A body-fat level of less than 11 percent can also be a sign of an eating disorder called anorexia nervosa.

For teenage males, less than 6 percent body fat is considered too low. Athletes, such as wrestlers, gymnasts, and dancers, should be especially careful to avoid too low a body-fat level. Even athletes should have at least the minimum amount of body fat. Medical research has shown that consistently low levels of body fat contribute to health problems. Some athletes mistakenly think that the lower their level of body fat, the better their performance in sports.

Though fewer males have anorexia nervosa than females, some do have this disorder. Teenage males also can be subject to a disorder called fear of obesity. This disorder is similar to, but less severe than, anorexia nervosa. A person with fear of obesity does not eat enough to maintain an ideal level of body fat. This condition can result in delayed maturity and ultimately being shorter than normal.

Females are considered overfat if more than 25 percent of their body weight is fat; over 35 percent fat is considered obese. Males are considered overfat if more than 20 percent of their body weight is fat; over 30 percent percentage is considered obese. The ideal—or optimal—amounts of body fat for good health and fitness are discussed later in this chapter.

Your body fatness can be determined by measuring the thickness of the fat under folds of skin. These folds are known as *skinfolds*, or *fatfolds*. A tool called *calipers* is used to measure skinfold thickness. When several skinfold measurements are added, the sum and a table can be used to estimate percentage of body fat.

Types of calipers

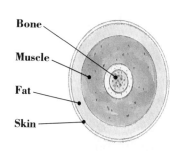

Bone
Muscle
Fat
Skin

Fat
Skin
Skinfold
Calipers

Measuring skinfold

NORMAL WEIGHT AND TARGET WEIGHT

Typical weight tables list the average weight range for people, according to age, height, and sex. You can use these tables to compare your weight to others your height, age, and sex. However, weight tables do not show body fat percentages.

Ideal weight, called *target weight*, is the one at which you have the proper amount of body fat. For your age group, males with less than 16 percent fat and females with less than 21 percent fat are at, or below, their target weights. Once you have learned your percentage of body fat, you might decide to lower your fat level for personal or performance reasons. However, be careful not to allow your percentage of body fat to get too low.

X rays, computers, and underwater weighing are among methods used to measure levels of body fat. These methods require special equipment and must be done by trained specialists. However, two methods of estimating body fatness—skinfold measurements and body measurements—do not take excessive time, equipment, or expertise.

Normal Weight Ranges

Males					Females				
Height Feet	Inches	Age 13–14	15–16	17–20	Height Feet	Inches	Age 13–14	15–16	17–20
4	6	69–72			4	6	73–76		
4	7	73–76			4	7	76–79		
4	8	78–81			4	8	79–82		
4	9	82–85	82–85		4	9	86–89	91–94	
4	10	87–90	87–90		4	10	91–94	98–101	99–102
4	11	88–91	88–91		4	11	96–909	102–105	104–107
5	0	89–92	97–100	101–104	5	0	104–107	106–109	109–112
5	1	97–100	101–104	106–109	5	1	105–108	109–112	113–116
5	2	100–103	106–109	114–117	5	2	106–109	112–115	116–119
5	3	106–109	111–114	121–124	5	3	110–113	115–118	120–123
5	3	113–116	115–118	124–127	5	4	115–118	120–123	125–128
5	5	116–119	120–123	129–132	5	5	119–122	124–127	129–132
5	6	120–123	126–129	134–137	5	6	126–129	128–131	134–137
5	7	126–129	132–135	137–140	5	7	127–130	131–134	137–140
5	8	130–133	135–138	140–143	5	8	128–131	135–138	143–146
5	9	135–138	139–142	147–150	5	9	129–132	137–140	148–151
5	10	141–144	142–145	149–152	5	10	130–133	139–142	153–156
5	11	146–149	149–152	152–155	5	11		142–145	158–161
6	0	151–154	152–155	156–159	6	0		146–149	163–166
6	1		158–161	162–165				146–149	163–166
6	2		160–163	167–170					
6	3 & over			177–180					

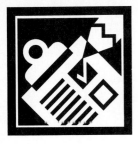

SELF-EVALUATION

IDENTIFYING TARGET WEIGHT

WORKSHEET 10-1

Record the results of your self-evaluation on worksheet 10-1.

Complete this self-evaluation to help you estimate your own percentage of body fat. Remember that each procedure takes practice and that your results are only an estimate of your body fat percentage.

PART 1: SKINFOLD MEASUREMENTS Skinfold measurements can be used to estimate body fat percentage and target weight. For teenagers, upper arm (triceps) and calf measurements provide a good estimate of fat percentage. Work with a partner to take each other's measurements. Record your findings on your worksheet.

● Triceps skinfold: Pick up a skinfold on the middle of the back of the right arm, halfway between the elbow and the shoulder. The arm should hang loose and relaxed at the side.

● Calf skinfold: Stand up and place your right foot on a chair. Pick up a skinfold on the side of your right calf half way between your shin and the back of your calf, where the calf is largest.

1. Use your left thumb and index finger to pick up the skinfold. Do not pinch or squeeze the skinfold.

2. Hold the skinfold with your left hand while holding the calipers with the right hand to get a reading.

3. Place the calipers over the skinfold about one-half inch below your finger and thumb. Hold the calipers on the skinfold for three seconds, and then note the measurement. Read the calipers measurement to the nearest one-half millimeter (mm), if possible.

4. Take 3 measurements each of the triceps and calf. Use the middle of the 3 measurements as your skinfold score. For example, an 8, 9, and 10 give a score of 9. If your 3 measurements differ by more than 2 mm, take a second, or even third, set of measurements.

5. Add the triceps and calf scores. Use the Skinfold Table to estimate your body-fat percentage. Then use a ruler to connect your sum of skinfolds with the percent fat figure. For example, if you are a male and your skinfolds' sum is 27 mm, then your body fat percentage is approximately 22%.

6. Next, turn to the Target Body Weight Tables on page 225. Find the row showing your body weight and the column with your estimated sum of skinfolds. Your target weight is where the columns intersect.

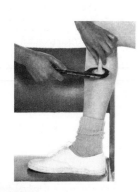

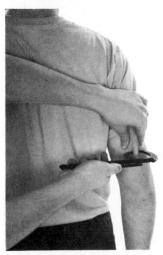

Measuring skinfold

Skinfold Measurements and Body Fat Percentages
(Sum of triceps plus calf skinfolds)

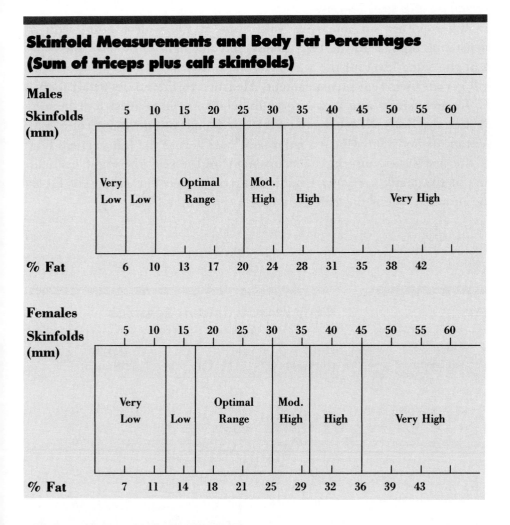

Males
Skinfolds (mm)

| 5 | 10 | 15 | 20 | 25 | 30 | 35 | 40 | 45 | 50 | 55 | 60 |

| Very Low | Low | Optimal Range | | Mod. High | High | | Very High |

% Fat

| 6 | 10 | 13 | 17 | 20 | 24 | 28 | 31 | 35 | 38 | 42 |

Females
Skinfolds (mm)

| 5 | 10 | 15 | 20 | 25 | 30 | 35 | 40 | 45 | 50 | 55 | 60 |

| Very Low | Low | Optimal Range | Mod. High | High | | Very High |

% Fat

| 7 | 11 | 14 | 18 | 21 | 25 | 29 | 32 | 36 | 39 | 43 |

Rating Chart: Body Fatness

Fitness Rating	% Fat (Males)
Too Little Fat	6 or less
High Performance	7–9
Good	10–19
Marginal	20–24
Too Much Fat	25 or more

Fitness Rating	% Fat (Females)
Too Little Fat	11 or less
High Performance	12–14
Good	15–24
Marginal	25–29
Too Much Fat	30 or more

PART 2: BODY MEASUREMENTS You can also use body measurements to estimate your percentage of body fat. One procedure uses weight and waist measurements for men and height and hip measurements for women. Follow the directions below. Work with a partner to take measurements. Record your results on your worksheet.

Males: Waist and Weight

1. Pull the measuring tape firmly, but not tightly, around your waist, even with your navel. Measure your waist to the nearest half inch.
2. Weigh yourself while fully clothed, but without shoes. Find your weight to the nearest pound.
3. Use the Body Measurement table to estimate your percentage of body fat. Place a ruler so that it cuts across the left vertical line at the mark for your weight and across the right vertical line at the mark for your waist measurement. Your estimated percentage of body fat is the number where the ruler intersects the slanted line.
4. Use the Target Body Weight table on page 225 to find your target weight. Then follow the procedure in step 6 of Skinfold Measurements.

Females: Hip and Height

1. With clothes on, measure your hips at the widest point with a measuring tape. Pull the tape firmly, but not tightly. Be sure the tape is at the same level all the way around your hips. If it is off line, you will get an incorrect measurement. Measure to the nearest half inch.

2. Remove shoes and measure your height to the nearest half inch.

3. Use the Body Measurement table for females to estimate your percentage of body fat. Place a ruler so it cuts across the left vertical line at the mark for your hip measurement and across the right vertical line at the mark for your height. Your estimated percentage of fat is the number where the ruler intersects the center line.

Body Measurement: Males

Body Weight (pounds)	% Fat	Waist (inches)
		45
120		
140	40	40
160	30	
	25	
180	20	35
200	15	
220	10	
240	5	30
260		
		25

Body Measurement: Females

Hip (inches)	% Fat	Height (inches)
32	10	
	14	72
34	18	70
		68
36	22	
	26	66
38	30	64
		62
40	34	
	38	60
42		58
	42	56

EXERCISE, WEIGHT GAIN, AND FAT LOSS

Most experts agree that a combination of exercise and proper diet regulation is best for controlling your level of body fat. Continue reading to learn how exercise and proper diet can help you lose body fat or gain weight, if necessary.

EXERCISE AND WEIGHT GAIN Proper exercise can increase muscle development in those individuals who want to gain weight. Since muscle weighs more than fat, exercise can produce dramatic results.

You already know that exercise or activity burns additional Calories. Therefore, an individual would have to consume more Calories than usual in order to gain weight. You do not have to eat a special diet to gain muscle; you only need to eat more of a well-balanced diet. If you increase the amount of food you eat without increasing your level of exercise, your added weight will be mainly fat. However, if your percentage of body fat is too low to begin with, some increase in body fat is not harmful.

EXERCISE AND FAT LOSS The U.S. Public Health Service studies show that overfatness and obesity are major health problems for many adults. The best way to avoid being overfat is to attain and maintain an ideal weight early in life.

A combination of exercise and a low-Calorie diet is the best way to lose body fat. Research shows that a person who reduces Calorie consumption without exercising might lose as much weight as a person who exercises and diets. However, the person who fails to exercise loses both fat and muscle. A person who both exercises and reduces Calorie consumption loses mostly body fat. A person who only exercises loses body fat, but not as rapidly as someone who both reduces Calorie consumption and exercises.

The best way to exercise is to find an activity that you enjoy. If you enjoy it, you are likely to exercise regularly. Physical activities of the type used for cardiovascular fitness are best for burning Calories for fat loss. Making exercise a regular part of your life is essential for controlling body fatness throughout your life, especially if you have inherited a tendency to have more body fat than normal.

CALORIES BURNED PER HOUR Every type of exercise burns some Calories. The more Calories burned while exercising, the more body fat is lost. The Energy Expenditure Table on page 130 shows the approximate number of Calories burned per hour during vigorous recreational play of activities, not from official competition or backyard play. It lists the approximate number of Calories burned per hour for a person who weighs 100 pounds, 120 pounds, 150 pounds, 180 pounds, or 200 pounds.

HAVE YOU HEARD?

Why do heavy people use up more Calories during exercise than lighter people do? According to physics, the heavier something is, the more energy it takes to move it from one place to another.

Find the weight value nearest your own weight. Add 5 percent to the number of Calories for each 10 pounds you weigh above the listed weight value. Or, subtract 5 percent from the number of Calories for each 10 pounds you weigh below the listed weight value. Use the Energy Expenditure Table to determine which physical activities are best for burning Calories. Then see which activities particularly appeal to you.

Energy Expenditure

Activity	Calories Used (per hour) Weight: 100 lbs.	120 lbs.	150 lbs.	180 lbs.	200 lbs.
Backpacking/Hiking	307	348	410	472	513
Badminton	255	289	340	391	425
Baseball	210	238	280	322	350
Basketball (half court)	225	225	300	345	375
Bicycling (normal speed)	157	178	210	242	263
Bowling	155	176	208	240	261
Canoeing (4 mph)	276	344	414	504	558
Circuit Training	247	280	330	380	413
Dance, Ballet	240	300	360	432	480
Dance, Aerobic	315	357	420	483	525
Dance, Modern	240	300	360	432	480
Dance, Social	174	222	264	318	348
Fencing	225	255	300	345	375
Fitness Calisthenics	232	263	310	357	388
Football	225	255	300	345	375
Golf (walking)	187	212	250	288	313
Gymnastics	232	263	310	357	388
Horseback Riding	180	204	240	276	300
Interval Training	487	552	650	748	833
Jogging (5$^{1}/_{2}$ mph)	487	552	650	748	833
Judo / Karate	232	263	310	357	388
Racquetball / Handball	450	510	600	690	750
Rope Jumping (continuous)	525	595	700	805	875
Rowing, Crew	615	697	820	943	1025
Running (10 m.p.h.)	625	765	900	1035	1125
Skating, Ice / Roller	262	297	350	403	438
Skiing, Cross-Country	525	595	700	805	875
Skiing, Downhill	450	510	600	690	750
Soccer	405	459	540	575	621
Softball (fast pitch)	210	238	280	322	350
Swimming (slow laps)	240	272	320	368	400
Swimming (fast laps)	420	530	630	768	846
Tennis	315	357	420	483	525
Volleyball	262	297	350	403	483
Walking	204	258	318	372	426
Waterskiing	306	390	468	564	636
Weight Training	352	399	470	541	558

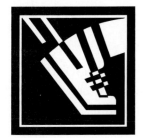

ACTIVITY

EXERCISING FOR FAT LOSS

You have learned how many Calories you might burn in one hour while performing certain exercises. Now use this activity to learn how effective different exercises are for controlling your level of body fat.

1. Choose two or more activities listed in this chart. During a 30-minute period, participate in the activities. Keep track of how much time you spend on each activity.

2. On your worksheet, record the name of each activity and the time you spent doing it. Determine how many Calories you probably used for each activity. Multiply the number of minutes you spent on each activity by the number of Calories used per minute, as shown on the chart. For example, if you spent 10 minutes walking briskly and weigh 150 pounds, you used about 5.3 Calories per minute. Ten minutes multiplied by 5.3 Calories equals 53 Calories.

3. Total your figures in the "Calories Used" column to find out how many Calories you probably burned in 30 minutes.

4. Recall that you must burn 3,500 Calories more than you consume to lose one pound of body fat. Divide 3,500 Calories by the number of Calories you used in the 30-minute exercise period to find out how many 30-minute exercise periods are needed to burn 3,500 Calories.

WORKSHEET 10-2

Use worksheet 10-2 to record your results of this activity.

Energy Expenditure

	Calories Used (per minute)					
Activity	Weight: less than 100	101– 125	126– 150	151– 175	176– 200	201– 225
Walking	2.3	2.9	3.5	4.1	4.7	5.2
Walking (brisk pace)	3.4	4.3	5.3	4.1	4.7	5.2
Fitness calisthenics	3.3	4.2	5.1	6.0	6.9	7.8
Badminton	3.7	4.7	5.7	6.7	7.7	8.7
Volleyball	3.8	4.8	5.8	6.8	7.8	8.8
Basketball (half court)	3.3	4.2	5.1	6.0	6.9	7.8
Jogging (12 minute mile)	7.1	9.0	10.8	12.6	14.5	16.4

MYTHS ABOUT EXERCISE AND FAT LOSS

Many people have three incorrect ideas about exercise and fat loss. First, some people mistakenly believe that exercise cannot be effective for fat loss because of the time it takes to use 3,500 Calories through exercise. For example, these people point out that a person has to play tennis for eight hours to lose one pound of fat. Since few individuals are likely to play tennis continuously for eight hours, these people mistakenly question the benefits of exercise for fat loss.

The fact is that you cannot lose large amounts of body fat quickly by exercising vigorously. However, you can lose body fat over a period of time with regular exercise if your Calorie intake remains the same. If you play one-half hour of tennis daily, you will lose 16 pounds in a year. Even walking makes a difference. If you briskly walk 15 minutes a day instead of watching TV, you will lose five to six pounds in a year. Thus, exercising is a good way to lose body fat over a period of time.

In addition, fat lost through exercise tends to stay off longer than fat lost by dieting alone. Weight lost by dieting alone is apt to include some loss of muscle as well as fat. Losing lean muscle tissue is not desirable. Exercise also prevents flabbiness.

The second mistaken belief is that exercise does not aid weight loss because it increases your appetite and encourages you to overeat. The fact is that your body cannot distinguish between inactivity and mild activity. Therefore, if you are mildly active instead of inactive, your appetite should not increase. Your appetite might increase from moderate and vigorous exercise, but not so much that you will overeat. People who overeat usually do so for reasons other than appetite.

Chapter 12 discusses other mistaken beliefs about fat loss, including the use of fad diets, useless weight-loss drugs, and ineffective exercise machines. Use this information to help design a plan that can help you lose excess body fat, gain muscle weight if you are underweight, or help you maintain your target weight.

Finally, some people mistakenly blame their overfat condition on a glandular problem. Only about five percent of overfat people have thyroid or other glandular problems that make controlling body fat levels difficult. The overwhelming majority of people are overfat because they eat too much or exercise too little or both.

Everyone has a different concept of the "ideal" figure or physique. Most people agree, however, that they would rather not be overfat. No matter what your body is like now, regular exercise and the proper diet will help you control body fatness. When you are lean and fit, you feel better, look better, and have fewer health problems than people who are unfit and overfat.

CHAPTER REVIEW

MULTIPLE CHOICE

Choose the letter of the best answer.

1. Which is *not* a function of body fat? (a) filter substances (b) shock absorber (c) insulator (d) stored energy

2. What do the words "overfat" and "underfat" describe? (a) amount of body fat (b) general build (c) muscle weight (d) bone size

3. One pound of body fat contains how many Calories? (a) 2,000 (b) 2,500 (c) 3,000 (d) 3,500

4. What advice should you give a friend who wants to lose weight in a hurry? (a) What you eat is less important than how much you eat. (b) Cut down on Calories. (c) Exercise regularly. (d) Cut down on Calories and exercise regularly.

5. A caliper measures (a) weight. (b) muscle length. (c) hip circumference. (d) skinfold thickness.

6. A female with 15 percent body fat is (a) underfat. (b) near target weight. (c) slightly overfat. (d) obese.

7. A male with 27 percent body fat is (a) underfat. (b) near target weight. (c) slightly overfat. (d) obese.

8. For women, which percentage of body fat is the minimum amount needed for good health? (a) 9 (b) 11 (c) 13 (d) 15

9. How many pounds per week can a person safely lose? (a) 1 to 2 (b) 2 to 3 (c) 3 to 4 (d) 4 to 5

10. Which method is best for losing body fat and maintaining the loss? (a) exercise only (b) lower Calorie consumption only (c) exercise and lower Calorie consumption combined (d) either exercise or lower Calorie consumption

11. Approximately how much body fat is located deep within your body? (a) 10% (b) 25% (c) 50% (d) 75%

MATCHING

Match the definition in Column I with the term it defines in Column II.

Column I

12. contains outer layer of fat
13. energy unit
14. refers to a very high percentage of body fat
15. having too little body fat
16. minimum amount needed for good health
17. ideal weight
18. person's eating habits

Column II

a. Calorie
b. diet
c. essential body fat
d. obesity
e. skinfold
f. target weight
g. underfat

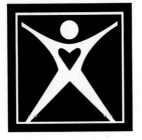

FOCUS ON FITNESS

AQUA DYNAMICS

Aqua dynamics is an exercise program performed in water. You perform exercises similar to those done outside of a pool. You also swim for brief periods of time.

Try this sample program. Note that even non-swimmers can use aqua dynamics. They should walk back and forth in waist- to chest-deep water for the "treading" and "lap swimming" parts of the program.

AQUA DYNAMICS

Exercise	Length of Time
Side Straddle Hop	15 seconds
Front Flutter	30 seconds
Back Flutter	30 seconds
Walking Twists	15 seconds
Toe Bounce	30 seconds
Pull and Stretch	30 seconds
Leg Out	30 seconds
Standing Crawl	30 seconds
Rearward Leg Bob	60 seconds
Leg Swing Out	30 seconds
Tread Water	1 minute
Lap Swimming (*Non-swimmers walk in water.*)	9 minutes

SIDE STRADDLE HOP

1. Stand in waist- to chest-deep water with hands on hips.
2. Jump sideways to position with feet 2 feet apart. Continue jumping for 15 seconds.

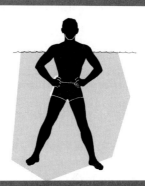

FRONT FLUTTER

1. Lie face down and hold on to the side of the pool.
2. Kick, flutter style, with your toes pointed back. Your ankles should be flexible and each knee straight, but not locked. Each leg acts as a whip.

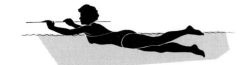

BACK FLUTTER

1. Lie on your back and hold onto the side of the pool.

2. Kick as described in Front Flutter.

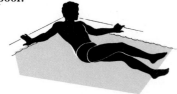

WALKING TWISTS

1. Clasp your hands behind your neck.
2. Walk forward, bringing your left leg up, and twisting your body to touch your left knee to your right elbow.
3. Repeat by bringing up your right leg and twisting your body to touch your right knee to your left elbow.

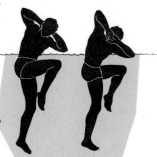

TOE BOUNCE

1. Stand in waist- to chest-deep water with hands on hips.
2. Jump high by pushing off with your feet together.

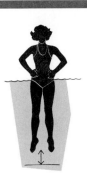

PULL AND STRETCH

1. Stand at the side of the pool with your back against the pool wall.
2. Raise your left leg, and grab under your left thigh with both arms. Pull your leg tightly to your chest.
3. Repeat with your right leg.

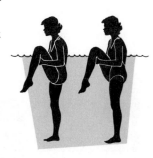

LEG OUT

1. Stand at the side of the pool with your back against the pool wall.
2. Raise your left knee to your chest.
3. Straighten your left leg out and stretch it. Drop your left leg to starting position.
4. Repeat with your right leg.

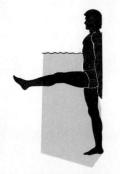

STANDING CRAWL

1. Stand in waist- to chest-deep water.
2. Reach out with your left hand and "grab" the water.
3. Press downward and pull. Bring your left hand through to your left thigh.
4. Repeat with your right hand and thigh.

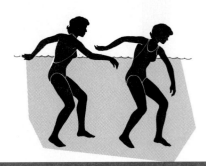

REARWARD LEG BOB

1. Stand in shallow water. Take a breath.
2. Sink under water with your left leg in squatting position. Your left foot should be on the pool bottom. Your right leg should be straight back. Breathe out while under water.
3. Shove off the bottom of the pool, and reverse the position of your legs. Take a breath when you surface.
4. Sink under water with your right leg in squatting position. Your left leg should be straight back. Repeat as described above.

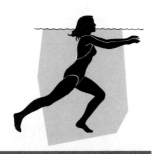

LEG SWING OUT

1. Stand with your back against the pool. Place your arms at shoulder height. Hold onto the pool gutter.
2. Raise your left leg in front of you as high as possible. Keep that leg straight.
3. Swing your leg to your left side. Pull the leg straight down as hard as possible.
4. Repeat with your right leg.

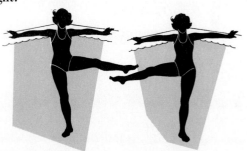

11

SKILL-RELATED FITNESS

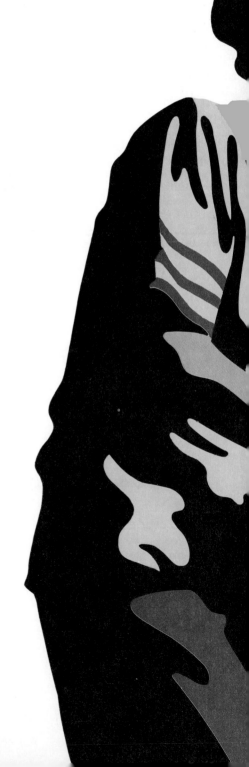

CHAPTER OBJECTIVES

After reading this chapter, you should be able to:

✔ Explain how skill-related fitness is related to good health.

✔ Determine how much skill-related fitness you need.

✔ Discuss how a person can learn sports skills.

You already know that physical fitness is divided into two categories: health-related fitness and skill-related fitness. The five parts of health-related fitness are considered the most important because you need them to maintain good health. A totally fit person, however, also has good skill-related fitness.

The six parts of skill-related fitness—agility, balance, coordination, power, speed, and reaction time—are related to performing well in sports and using physical skills. In this chapter, you will learn about the importance of each part of skill-related fitness. You will also learn how to evaluate and improve your own skill-related fitness. Above all, you will see how the improvement of this area of fitness can be fun.

WHAT IS SKILL-RELATED FITNESS?

Skills are specific physical tasks that people can perform, such as catching, throwing, swimming, batting, and dancing. You learned in Chapter 1 that *skill-related fitness* is a group of basic abilities that help you learn particular skills. Notice that physical skills and skill-related fitness are not the same. For example, you can develop your balance and coordination (two parts of skill-related fitness) to improve the skill of swinging a bat. Several factors affect the level of skill-related fitness a person can attain. These factors include heredity, practice, and the principle of specificity.

HEREDITY Medical evidence has shown that parts of skill-related fitness, such as speed and reaction time, are greatly influenced by heredity. Some people are able to run fast or react quickly because they inherited these traits from their parents. If you did not inherit a tendency to excel in these areas, it may be more difficult for you to perform skills that require those abilities. It is never impossible, however, to improve skills, and often extra practice and desire make up for a lack of "natural" ability.

PRACTICE While skill-related fitness is needed to learn specific skills, you still must practice to improve those skills. Practice is what helps you improve skills such as hitting a tennis ball or batting a baseball. While everyone cannot become an Olympic athlete, all people can learn the basic skills necessary to enjoy sports and to perform physical tasks efficiently. Practice is the key!

PRINCIPLE OF SPECIFICITY The principle of specificity applies to skill-related fitness as well as health-related fitness. Keep in mind that just because you might excel in one part of skill-related fitness, you will not necessarily excel in other parts. This is often the case even regarding abilities that seem closely related, such as reaction time and speed. For example, you might have great speed, which helps your skill of running down fly balls in the outfield during softball. But poor reaction time prevents you from getting a good "jump" on the ball. In this case, you might choose a sport or activity that emphasizes speed rather than reaction time.

BENEFITS OF SKILL-RELATED FITNESS

Developing and maintaining skill-related fitness influences your health. People who use skill-related fitness to improve their skills in sports and games are more likely to be physically active than those who do not have these skills. As a result, active people are more likely to improve their health through exercise. In addition, people who learn skills gain two other important benefits: they generally enjoy life and feel good about themselves. Perhaps you have had the experience of being uneasy at a dance because you felt you did not dance well. People generally enjoy doing things they do well. Improving your skill-related fitness is a first big step toward improving those skills that will help you enjoy life and improve your self-image.

This chapter's self-evaluations will give you an idea of the parts of skill-related fitness you do best. Then you can determine which parts you would like to improve. This information also could help you select recreational activities that use the abilities you already have.

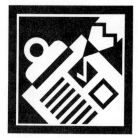

SELF-EVALUATION

BALANCE, COORDINATION, AND REACTION TIME

Use this self-evaluation to evaluation your balance, coordination, and reaction time. Keep these points in mind, especially if you score low:

- You can improve all parts of your skill-related fitness.
- Many activities do not require high levels of these abilities.
- You need not excel in an activity to enjoy it.

BALANCE You need a 2″ x 2″ stick 1 foot long for these tests. Wear gym shoes while taking these tests. Record your scores on your worksheet. You may take 1 practice try before taking each test for a score.

WORKSHEET 11-1

Use worksheet 11-1 to record your results of this self-evaluation.

Test 1

1. Place balls of both feet across the stick so that your heels are on the floor.
2. Lift your heels off the floor and maintain your balance on the stick for 15 seconds. Keep your arms held out straight in front of you. Do not allow your heels to touch the floor or your feet to move on the stick once you begin.
3. Test yourself twice. Give yourself 2 points if you are successful on the first try, 1 point if you failed on the first try, but succeeded on the second, and 3 points if you were successful on both tries. Try test 2 even if you did not do well on test 1.

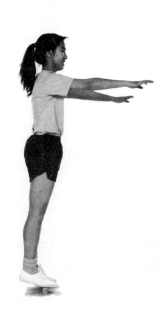

Test 2

1. Stand on the stick with either your left foot or right foot. Your foot should run the length of the stick.
2. Lift your other foot off the floor. First, balance for 10 seconds with your foot flat. Then rise up on your toes and continue balancing for 10 seconds.
3. Test yourself twice. Give yourself 1 point if you balanced for 10 seconds flat-footed, and another point if you balanced on your toes for 10 seconds. Give yourself another point if you successfully balanced both flat-footed and standing on your toes. Your maximum score is 3 points.

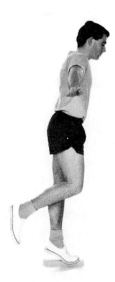

COORDINATION You need three 24″ dowel rods (1/2″ diameter) for this test. Take three practice tries before taking the test for a score.

1. Hold a stick in each hand. Have a partner put a third stick across your sticks.
2. Toss the third stick in the air so that it makes a half turn. Catch it with the sticks you are holding. The tossed stick should not hit your hands.

3. Take this test 5 times tossing the stick to the right, and 5 times tossing to the left. Score 1 point for each successful catch.

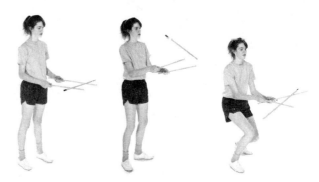

REACTION TIME You need a yardstick and a partner for this test.

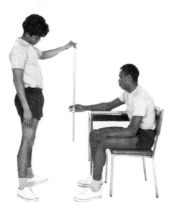

1. Have your partner hold the top of the yardstick with the thumb and index finger between the 1-inch mark and the end of the yardstick.
2. Position your thumb and fingers at the 24-inch mark on the yardstick. Your thumb and fingers should *not* touch the yardstick. Your arm should rest on the edge of a table with only your hand over the edge.
3. When your partner drops the stick without warning, catch it as quickly as possible between your thumb and fingers. Your score is the number on the yardstick at which you caught it.
4. Try this test 3 times. Your partner should be careful not to drop the yardstick after the same waiting period each time. You should not be able to guess when the yardstick will drop.

SCORING AND RATING After recording your individual test scores and total scores on your worksheet, find your *total score* for each test on the rating chart. Record your rating on your worksheet. In class, you might only have time to take each test once. However, try to retest yourself periodically. You might save your worksheet and use it to record future test results so you can note your progress.

Rating Chart: Balance, Coordination, and Reaction Time*

Performance Rating	Balance Test	Coordination Test	Reaction Time Test
High	6	9 to 10	more than 21 inches
Good	5	7 to 8	19 to 21 inches
Marginal	3 to 4	4 to 6	14 to 18 ³/₄ inches
Low	less than 3	less than 4	less than 14 inches

*Note: Since skill-related fitness does not relate directly to good health, the "good fitness" rating is not used.

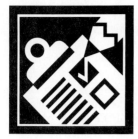

SELF-EVALUATION

AGILITY, POWER, AND SPEED

Use this self-evaluation to evaluate your agility, power, and speed.

AGILITY Use masking tape or other materials to make five parallel lines on the floor, each three feet apart. Have a partner count while you take the test. Then count while your partner takes the test.

1. Stand with both feet to the left of the line at the far left. When your partner says "go," slide to the right until your right foot steps outside the far right line. Then slide to the left until your left foot steps outside the far left line. *Note:* Be careful not to cross your feet.
2. Repeat, moving right-to-left and back, as many times as possible in 10 seconds. Only 1 foot must cross the outside lines.
3. When your partner says "stop," freeze in place until your partner counts your score. Score 1 point for each line you crossed in 10 seconds. Subtract 1 point for each time you crossed your feet.
4. Take this test twice. Record the better of your 2 scores on your worksheet.

WORKSHEET 11-2

Use worksheet 11-2 to record your results of this self-evaluation.

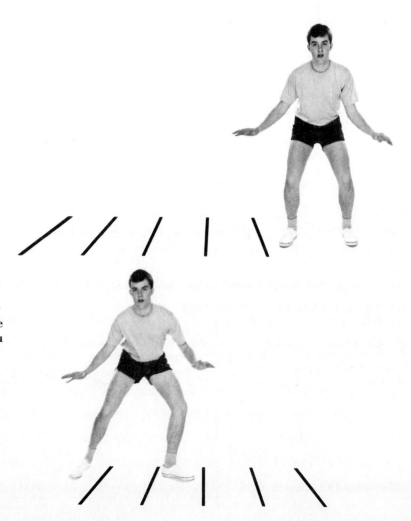

POWER Use masking tape or other materials to make a line on the floor. You also need a tape measure.

1. Stand with both feet behind the line on the floor. Swing your arms forward, and jump as far as possible. Keep both feet together. Do not run or hop before jumping.

2. Have a partner measure the distance from the line to the

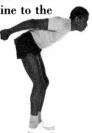

nearest point where any part of your body touched the floor when you landed.

3. Take this test twice. Record the better of your 2 scores on your worksheet.

SPEED You need a stopwatch, a whistle, and a specially marked running course to take this test. Use masking tape or other material to make lines 2 yards apart starting 10 yards from the starting line for a total distance of 26 yards. Work with a partner who will time you with the stopwatch and blow the whistle to signal you to stop.

Try this test once for practice without being timed; then try it for a score. Record your score on your worksheet.

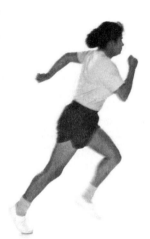

1. Stand 2 or 3 steps behind the starting line. Your partner will start the stopwatch when you cross the starting line.
2. When your partner says "go," run as far and as fast as you can

until your partner blows the whistle 3 seconds later. Do not try to stop immediately, but begin to slow down *after* the whistle blows.
3. Your partner will mark where you were

when the whistle blew. Measure the distance to the nearest yard line. Your score is the distance you covered in the 3 seconds *after* crossing the starting line.

SCORING AND RATING After recording your individual test scores on your worksheet, find your scores on the rating chart. Record your ratings on your worksheet.

Rating Chart: Agility, Power, and Speed*

Performance Rating	Agility (lines crossed)		Power (inches jumped)		Speed (yards run)	
	Males	**Females**	**Males**	**Females**	**Males**	**Females**
High	31 or more	28 or more	87 or more	74 or more	24 or more	22 or more
Good	26–30	24–27	80–86 in.	66–73 in.	21–23 yds	19–21 yds
Marginal	19–25	16–23	70–79	58–65	17–20	15–18
Low	less than 19	less than 15	less than 70	less than 58	less than 16	less than 15

*Note: Since skill-related fitness does not relate directly to good health, the "good fitness" rating is not used.

IMPROVING SKILL-RELATED FITNESS

You can improve a specific part of skill-related fitness by practicing activities that use that part of fitness. The chart on page 144 shows which activities are best for each part of skill-related fitness.

AGILITY *Agility* is the ability to change your body position quickly and to control your body's movements. It is an important factor in activities such as gymnastics, basketball, soccer, and modern dance.

BALANCE *Balance* is the ability to keep an upright posture while standing still or moving. Standing or walking on a line or a beam, or balancing objects in your hands or on your head are activities that help improve balance. It is a contributing factor in activities such as ballet, springboard or platform diving, and some areas of gymnastics.

COORDINATION *Coordination* is the ability to use your senses together with your body parts. You can improve different kinds of cordination, such as eye-hand and eye-foot coordination, by practicing the skill you want to learn. For example, basketball players would practice shooting and dribbling to improve hand-eye coordination. Remember to practice skills using both the right and left sides of your body.

POWER *Power* is the ability to use strength quickly. It is the part of skill-related fitness most likely to improve with repeated effort. You can improve your power by using the exercises in Chapter 7. However, strength exercises alone might not build optimal power. The strongest people are not necessarily the most powerful. New exercises have been developed for people interested in developing power for high-level performance. If you are interested in developing power, consult your instructor or coach for more information.

SPEED *Speed* is the ability to perform a movement or cover a distance in a short period of time. If you are not very strong, you might build up your strength to increase speed. You might also learn the best way to move for a particular activity, and then practice those movements.

REACTION TIME *Reaction time* is the amount of time it takes you to move once you realize the need to act. Practice helps reaction time because you learn what to react to and when to react. For example, sprinters can learn to react faster to the starting gun.

HAVE YOU HEARD?

The skills of the archer have been celebrated in story and song throughout history. Today archery is one of the most interesting activities available, and many types of archery competition exist. For example, in archery golf, the object is to hit a small target near a putting green in as few shots as possible.

LEARNING SPORTS SKILLS

Use these suggestions to improve your sports skills:

- **Get correct instruction.** If you learn a skill incorrectly, it will be hard to improve, even with practice.
- **Do not worry about details.** When you first learn a skill, concentrate on the skill as a whole, not its details. Details can be dealt with after the main skill is learned.
- **Keep practicing.** Many people do not like to practice skills; they just want to "play the game." However, just playing the game does not provide practice for a particular skill. Also, when you play a game without having the proper skills, you often develop bad habits that hinder your success and enjoyment of the game.
- **Avoid competition when learning a skill.** While competition can be fun, competing when you are learning a skill might be stressful.
- **Choose an activity that matches your skill-related fitness.** Learn an activity that uses the parts of skill-related fitness that you possess. This chart lists skill-related benefits for many activities. Use worksheet 11-3 to help you choose activities that best suit your abilities.

WORKSHEET 11-3

Use worksheet 11-3 to help you choose activities that best suit your abilities.

Skill-Related Benefits of Sports and Other Activities

Activity	Balance	Coordination	Reaction Time	Agility	Power	Speed
Badminton	Fair	Excellent	Good	Good	Fair	Good
Baseball	Good	Excellent	Excellent	Good	Excellent	Good
Basketball	Good	Excellent	Excellent	Excellent	Excellent	Good
Bicycling	Excellent	Fair	Fair	Poor	Poor	Fair
Bowling	Good	Excellent	Poor	Fair	Fair	Fair
Circuit Training	Fair	Fair	Poor	Fair	Good	Fair
Dance, Aerobic/Social	Fair	Good	Fair	Good	Poor	Poor
Dance, Ballet/Modern	Excellent	Excellent	Fair	Excellent	Good	Poor
Fitness Calisthenics	Fair	Fair	Poor	Good	Fair	Poor
Football	Good	Good	Excellent	Excellent	Excellent	Excellent
Golf (walking)	Fair	Excellent	Poor	Fair	Good	Poor
Gymnastics	Excellent	Excellent	Good	Excellent	Excellent	Fair
Interval Training	Fair	Fair	Poor	Poor	Poor	Fair
Jogging/Walking	Fair	Fair	Poor	Poor	Poor	Poor
Judo/Karate	Good	Excellent	Excellent	Excellent	Excellent	Excellent
Racquetball/Handball	Fair	Excellent	Good	Excellent	Fair	Good
Rope Jumping	Fair	Good	Fair	Good	Fair	Poor
Skating, Ice/Roller	Excellent	Good	Fair	Good	Fair	Good
Skiing, Cross-Country	Fair	Excellent	Poor	Good	Excellent	Fair
Skiing, Downhill	Excellent	Excellent	Good	Excellent	Good	Poor
Soccer	Fair	Excellent	Good	Excellent	Good	Good
Softball (fast pitch)	Fair	Excellent	Excellent	Good	Good	Good
Swimming (laps)	Fair	Good	Poor	Good	Fair	Poor
Tennis	Fair	Excellent	Good	Good	Good	Good
Volleyball	Fair	Excellent	Good	Good	Fair	Fair
Weight Training	Fair	Fair	Poor	Poor	Fair	Poor

CHAPTER REVIEW

MULTIPLE CHOICE

Choose the letter of the best answer.

1. Which is *not* a part of skill-related fitness? (a) agility (b) speed (c) power (d) weight

2. The parts of skill-related fitness are (a) not needed for overall fitness. (b) skills needed for sports. (c) abilities that help you learn sports skills. (d) all related to strength.

3. Inherited traits (a) make it easier or harder for you to develop certain skills. (b) do not affect your ability to develop skills. (c) come from one parent only. (d) make it impossible to develop many skills.

4. If you excel in one particular part of skill-related fitness, you (a) excel at all parts of skill-related fitness. (b) excel at all parts of health-related fitness. (c) might not excel at others. (d) cannot excel at others.

5. Most sports and activities require (a) superior speed. (b) only one part of skill-related fitness. (c) two or more parts of skill-related fitness. (d) good ratings in all parts of skill-related fitness.

6. Which is a skill? (a) balance (b) diving (c) speed (d) agility

7. You can best improve your skill-related fitness by (a) cutting down on fats. (b) eating a variety of foods. (c) building up your muscular endurance. (d) practicing.

8. When first learning a skill, you should (a) concentrate on the general skill. (b) concentrate on the skill's details. (c) practice the skill only twice. (d) compete.

9. To learn sports skills, first (a) learn the skills while playing the game in which they are used. (b) learn an incorrect way of doing the skills. (c) learn the skills correctly so you do not have to unlearn them later. (d) choose skills for which you have little skill-related fitness.

10. By developing and maintaining skill-related fitness, you are more likely to (a) have poor health-related fitness. (b) have good health-related fitness. (c) have a poor self-image. (d) be physically inactive.

MATCHING

Match the definition in Column I with the term it defines in Column II.

Column I

11. amount of time it takes you to move once you realize need to move
12. ability to keep an upright posture while standing still or moving
13. using senses together with body parts
14. ability to use strength quickly
15. ability to change body position quickly

Column II

a. agility
b. balance
c. coordination
d. power
e. reaction time

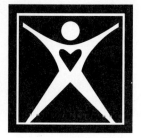

JUMP-ROPE WORKOUT

Jump-rope has become a popular exercise for all ages. It improves health-related, as well as skill-related, fitness. Athletes often jump rope to improve their cardiovascular fitness and coordination.

Before beginning a jump-rope workout, learn some of the skills associated with the activity. Some of the skills are simple, while others are more difficult. This workout includes only basic jump-rope skills. Add other, more difficult skills as your ability improves. As with any activity, using correct technique reduces your risk of injury. Keep these guidelines in mind:

● Start out slowly if you do not do jumping exercises regularly. Repeated bouncing can make your legs sore.

● Since jumping rope uses mostly leg muscles, your legs might fatigue after only a few minutes of exercise. Take periodic breaks to rest your legs. While resting, do stretching exercises or walk in a circle to help reduce leg soreness.

JUMP ROPE WORKOUT

Exercise	Rate of Jumping (turns per minute)	Length of Time or Repetitions	Exercise	Rate of Jumping (turns per minute)	Length of Time or Repetitions
Jog Step	120	1 minute	Two Foot Hop	130	1 minute
Left Side Swing	120	1 minute	Left Side Swing	120	1 minute
Right Side Swing	120	1 minute	Right Side Swing	120	1 minute
Calf Stretcher		3 each leg	Back Saver Toe Touch		3
Left Foot Hop	130	½ minute	Two-Foot Alternate		
Right Foot Hop	130	½ minute	High Hop	90	1 minute
Jog Step	120	1 minute	Jog Step	120	1 minute
Rest (walk in circle)		2 minutes			

JOG STEP

Jump from one foot, then the other foot.

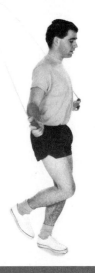

LEFT- OR RIGHT-FOOT HOP

Hop on your left or right foot with each rope swing. Beginners should hop twice for each rope swing.

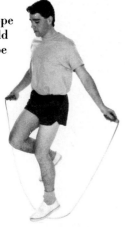

LEFT- OR RIGHT-SIDE SWING

Swing the rope to your left or right side as you jump beside it.

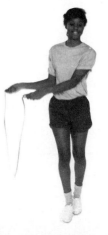

TWO-FOOT HOP
TWO-FOOT ALTERNATE HIGH HOP

1. Hop on both feet with each rope swing. Beginners should hop twice with each rope swing.
2. For two-foot alternate high hop, lift your knees high for every other hop.

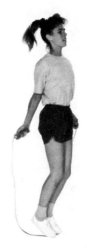

CALF STRETCHER

● See page 10 for directions for this exercise.

BACK SAVER TOE TOUCH

● See page 115 for directions for the back saver toe touch.

OTHER SKILLS As you become better at jump rope, you might want to try these more advanced skills:
● **One-foot Double** The one-foot double is performed the same way as the one-foot hop except that you swing the rope twice for each hop.
● **Two-foot Double** The two-foot double is performed the same way as the two-foot hop except that you swing the rope twice for each hop.
● **Cross Swing** The cross swing is performed the same way as the two-foot hop except that you cross your arms every other time you swing the rope.

12

NUTRITION

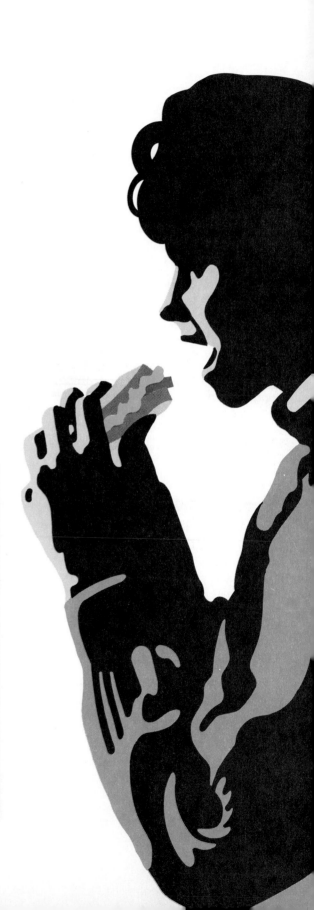

CHAPTER OBJECTIVES

After reading this chapter, you should be able to:

✔ Name sources of each of the six nutrient groups.

✔ List examples of foods in each of the four food groups.

✔ Name foods that you should eat only in limited quantities.

✔ Discuss eating disorders and the health problems they can cause.

✔ Discuss how to maintain a balanced, healthful diet.

You will look and feel your best if you eat right and get plenty of exercise. Nevertheless, studies show that the majority of teenagers tend to eat many of the wrong kinds of foods, skip meals, and use unhealthful weight-reduction diets.

COMMON FOOD MYTHS

You probably have heard a number of incorrect or misleading statements about nutrition, such as the ones listed here:

- *Myth:* **Athletes need a steak, "high-energy" drink, or food supplement before they compete.** Many athletes mistakenly think that the demands of a sport require a special diet. A number of fad diets and dietary supplements have been developed especially for athletes. None of these measures is necessary. On the other hand, athletes who are training or competing should increase their Calorie intake. For their extra Calories, they should choose foods that are very nutritious.

- *Myth:* **Honey is more nutritious than sugar.** Chemically, honey is quite like refined sugar. Honey contains a few other nutritious substances, but they are not in large enough amounts to be of any benefit. You should limit your use of sugars, including honey.

- *Myth:* **Foods labeled "natural" or "organic" are more nutritious than other foods.** Often, such foods are not actually very nutritious. For example, some of the so-called "natural" granola-type cereals contain as much sugar and fat as other cereals.

- *Myth:* **A poor diet causes acne and other skin problems.** Food allergies can cause skin problems, but most skin problems are caused by rapid changes in hormones that occur during adolecsence. Hormones control oil glands, which can be very active during teenage years. Anxiety and emotional stress can aggravate to this problem.

This chapter cannot present a complete list of incorrect ideas such as the ones above, but it will discuss the basic principles of *nutrition—* the study of foods and how they nourish the body. You will also learn how to use those principles to plan a healthful diet.

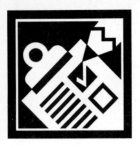

SELF-EVALUATION

NUTRITION KNOWLEDGE

WORKSHEET 12-1

Use Worksheet 12-1 to find out what you know about nutrition.

Use this self-evaluation to find out what you know about nutrition. Answer the questions on worksheet 12-1. Check your answers against the correct answers provided by your instructor. Total your correct answers and record the number on your worksheet. Check your score on the rating chart to see how you rate on your knowledge of nutrition. Record your rating on the worksheet.

NUTRIENTS YOUR BODY NEEDS

Scientists have identified 45 to 50 different *nutrients*—food substances required for the growth and maintenance of your cells. These nutrients have been divided into six groups—carbohydrates, proteins, fats, vitamins, minerals, and water. By eating the right amounts of foods containing these nutrient groups, you should get a balanced, healthful diet. The six groups are described here.

Rating Chart: Nutrition Knowledge

Rating	Correct Answers
High	18–20
Good	16–17
Marginal	14–15
Low	13 or less

CARBOHYDRATES *Carbohydrates* are nutrients that provide you with energy. Many foods are sources of carbohydrates. S*imple carbohydrates*, such as fruits, milk, molasses, and honey, are sugars that can be used by your body with little or no change during digestion. Breads, vegetables, and grains are examples of *complex carbohydrates*—foods that contain more of the other nutrients than do simple carbohydrates. Thus, you receive the benefits of a variety of nutrients by eating complex carbohydrates. Such foods are considered *nutritionally dense*, meaning they contain large amounts of nutrients for the number of Calories they provide.

Simple carbohydrates

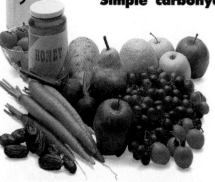

Complex carbohydrates

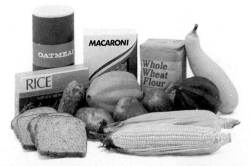

Fiber is a type of carbohydrate that your body cannot digest. Therefore, fiber supplies no energy. Fiber sources include the leaves, stems, roots, and seed coverings of fruits, vegetables, and grains. Some examples of foods high in fiber content are whole-wheat and whole-grain breads, unskinned fresh fruits, raw vegetables, nuts, and seeds. Fiber in your diet provides bulk that aids in eliminating wastes. Fiber also helps you avoid intestinal problems, and might reduce your chances of developing some forms of cancer.

PROTEIN *Proteins* are the building blocks of your body. The cells in your body are made of proteins. Foods containing proteins come from animal products, such as milk, eggs, meat, and fish. In addition, some plants, such as beans and grains, are good sources of proteins.

Proteins are composed of even smaller building blocks, called *amino acids*. Combinations of 22 kinds of amino acids form hundreds of different types of proteins. During digestion, your body breaks proteins down into amino acids, which your small intestine can absorb. Cells in the human body can manufacture 14 of the 22 amino acids. People get the other eight amino acids—known as the *essential amino acids*—from the foods they eat.

Foods with all eight essential amino acids are said to contain *complete proteins*. Complete proteins come from animal sources, such as meat, milk products, and fish. Foods that contain some, but not all, essential amino acids are said to contain *incomplete proteins*. Sources of incomplete proteins are beans, nuts, rice, and certain other plants. A daily diet that includes foods with both complete and incomplete proteins usually provides ample essential amino acids. People who regularly eat meats, fish, poultry, eggs, and milk products probably are getting enough proteins. People who do not eat meat, or those who are trying to lose weight, should make sure they include enough complete proteins in their diets.

FATS Like carbohydrates, *fats* provide energy. However, ounce for ounce, fats provide twice as much energy as carbohydrates do. Fats are major constituents in animal products and in some plant products, such as nuts and vegetable oils.

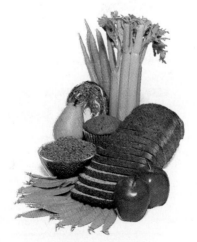

Foods rich in fiber

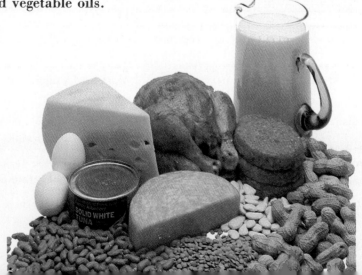

Sources of protein

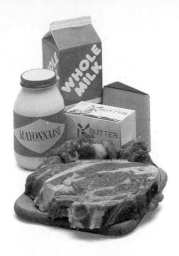

Sources of saturated fats

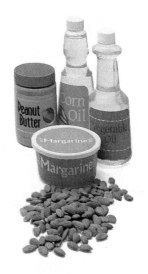

Sources of unsaturated fats

Fats have many important functions in the human body. They are necessary for the growth and repair of cells. Fats dissolve certain vitamins and carry them to the cells where they are needed. In addition, fats enhance the flavor and texture of foods. For instance, fats are responsible for the appetizing aroma of roast beef.

Because of differences in chemical structure, fats are classified as saturated or unsaturated. In general, *saturated fats* are solid at room temperature; *unsaturated fats* are liquid at room temperature. Saturated fats come mostly from animal products, such as lard, butter, milk, and meat fats. Unsaturated fats come mostly from plants, such as sunflowers, corn, soybeans, olives, almonds, and peanuts. Also, fish produce unsaturated fats in their cells.

Cholesterol is a waxy, fat-like substance found in the saturated fats of animal cells, including those of humans. You not only produce your own cholesterol, you consume cholesterol in certain foods. Some people have abnormally high levels of cholesterol that can contribute to atherosclerosis and other heart diseases. Medical experts recommend limiting cholesterol in your daily diet by eating foods low in cholesterol and low in saturated fat.

MINERALS *Minerals* are nutrients that perform many different functions in regulating the activities of cells. Minerals have no Calories and provide no energy. However, small amounts of minerals are essential for good health.

Minerals come from elements in the earth's crust. They are present in all plants and animals. The table shows some major functions of minerals and food sources in which important minerals are concentrated in usable amounts.

Functions and Sources of Minerals

Minerals	Function in the body	Food sources
Calcium	Builds and maintains teeth and bones; helps blood clot; helps nerves and muscles function	Cheese; milk; dark green vegetables; sardines; legumes
Phosphorus	Builds and maintains teeth and bones; helps release energy from nutrients	Meat; poultry; fish; eggs; legumes; milk products
Magnesium	Aids breaking down of glucose and proteins, regulates body fluids	Green vegetables; grains; nuts; beans; yeast
Sodium	Regulates internal water balance; helps nerves function	Most foods; table salt
Potassium	Regulates fluid balance in cells; helps nerves function	Oranges; bananas; meats; bran; potatoes; dried beans
Iron	Helps transfer oxygen in red blood cells and in other cells	Liver; red meats; dark green vegetables; shellfish; whole-grain cereals
Zinc	Aids in transport of carbon dioxide; aids in healing wounds	Meats; shellfish; whole grains; milk; legumes

VITAMINS *Vitamins* are needed for growth and repair of body cells. Like minerals, vitamins do not contain Calories and provide no energy. Some vitamins are water soluble; others are soluble only in fat. These factors are important since body fluids are watery solutions.

Vitamin C and the B vitamins dissolve in blood and are carried to cells throughout your body. Excess B and C vitamins are eliminated from your body in urine. Thus, your body cannot "store" these vitamins for use later. As a result, you should eat foods containing vitamins B and C every day. Vitamins A, D, E, and K dissolve in fat rather than water. When more of these vitamins are consumed than are needed, the excess amounts are stored in fat cells in your liver and other parts of your body.

Taking too much of a vitamin supplement can cause vitamins to accumulate in your body. Even water-soluble vitamins are toxic, or poisonous, if taken in large amounts. Vitamin buildups have been known to cause liver damage and other serious health problems. The table gives more information about vitamins.

HAVE YOU HEARD?

Your body needs only trace amounts of all vitamins and most minerals daily. However, larger amounts of a few minerals are required. For example, larger amounts of calcium and potassium are needed to build and maintain bones and teeth.

Functions and Sources of Vitamins

Vitamins	Function in the body	Food sources
B1 (Thiamin)	Helps release energy from carbohydrates	Pork; organ meats; legumes; greens
B2 (Riboflavin)	Helps breakdown carbohydrates, and proteins	Meat; milk products; eggs; green and yellow vegetables
B6 (Pyridoxine)	Helps breakdown protein and glucose	Yeast; nuts; beans; liver; fish; rice
B12 (Cobalamin)	Aids nucleic acid and amino acid formation	Meat; milk products; eggs; fish
Folacin	Helps build DNA and proteins	Yeast; wheat germ; liver; greens
Pantothenic acid	Involved in reactions with carbohydrates, and proteins	Most unprocessed foods
Niacin	Helps release energy from carbohydrates, and proteins	Milk; meats; whole-grain or enriched cereals; legumes
Biotin	Aids formation of amino, nucleic, and fatty acids and glycogen	Eggs; liver; yeast
C (Absorbic acid)	Aids formation or hormones, bone tissue, and collagen	Fruits, tomatoes; potatoes; green, leafy vegetables
A (Retinol)	Helps produce normal mucus, part of chemical necessary for vision	Butter; margarine; liver; eggs; green or yellow vegetables
D	Aids absorption of calcium and phosphorous	Liver; fortified milk; fatty fish
E (Tocopherol)	Prevents damage to cell membranes and vitamin A	Vegetable oils
K	Aids blood blotting	Leafy vegetables

WATER Water is the single most important nutrient. You can live for some time without the other nutrients, but you cannot live more than a few days without water. Water makes up a large percentage of all the foods you eat and beverages you drink. Your own body weight is 60 to 70 percent water.

You lose two to three quarts of water a day by perspiring, eliminating, and breathing. In very hot weather, or when you exercise vigorously, you may lose even more. The water lost must be replaced by water in foods and beverages.

Water has many life-sustaining functions in the body. For example, it carries nutrients to cells and removes wastes from cells. Water helps regulate your body temperature. The water in body fluids is needed for the chemical reactions that continuously take place in cells.

PLANNING A BALANCED DIET

A balanced, healthful diet includes proper amounts of the six nutrients. Food scientists have developed a guideline, called the *United States Recommended Daily Allowances (U.S. RDA)*. This guideline lists the recommended daily nutritional requirements for people, according to sex, age, height, and weight. The U.S. RDA gives the daily requirements for vitamins, minerals, proteins and Calories. The nutrient requirements are listed in grams or fractions of grams.

THE FOUR FOOD GROUPS Food scientists also have provided a relatively easy way to plan a balanced diet. By eating the daily recommended number of servings from each of four food groups, you should get enough of all the nutrients for a balanced, healthful diet.

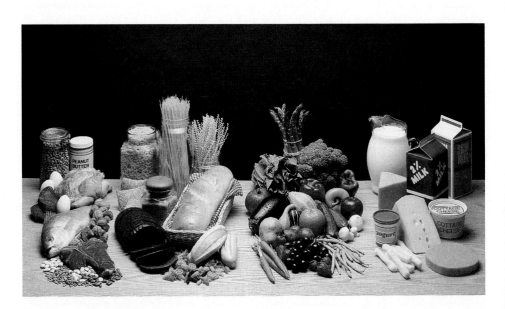

The four food groups

The *four food groups* are the meat-poultry-fish-bean group, bread-cereal group, fruit-vegetable group, and milk group. The group to which a food belongs depends on the nutrients it contains and its source. For example, foods in the bread-cereal group provide carbohydrates and come from plants.

The table shows examples of some foods in each of the four food groups and the recommended serving sizes of each. When selecting foods, be sure to include a variety of foods from within each group. Eating only one kind of fruit or vegetable day after day cannot provide all the vitamins and minerals you need.

Notice that jams, jellies, syrups, candies, soft drinks, and most commercially prepared snack foods do not appear in the four food groups. Most people eat some "extra foods" of this type, but these foods are not necessary for good health. These extra foods often contain fats, salt, and simple carbohydrates, but little else. Medical experts recommend cutting down on these foods or avoiding them.

HAVE YOU HEARD?

"Fast foods" are often high in fat, salt and Calories. A typical fast-food cheeseburger, french fries, and 12-ounce chocolate shake can contain 1,200 Calories, or half of your daily Calorie need. This meal also contains about 56 grams of fat and about 1/10 gram (100 mg) of sodium.

Using the Four Food Groups

	Food	Serving Size
Meat-Poultry-Fish-Bean Group 2 servings/day	bean, meat, poultry, or fish	2 or 3 ounces cooked
	eggs	2
	legumes (beans or peas)	1 cup cooked
	peanut butter	4 tablespoons
	nuts or sunflower seeds	2 ounces
Fruit-Vegetable Group 4 servings/day	potato	1 medium size
	orange	1
	cooked vegetable	1 ½ cup
	fruit juice	½ cup
	cooked fruit	½ cup
Bread-Cereal Group 4 servings/day	whole-grain wheat bread	1 slice
	cooked cereal	½ cup
	ready-to-eat cereal	1 cup
	cooked rice	½ cup
	wheat germ	¼ cup
	cooked pasta	½ cup
	tortilla	1 6-inch
Milk Group 4 servings/day	milk or yogurt	1 cup
	cottage cheese	½ cup
	cheese	2 ounces
	ice cream or ice milk	1-¾ cup

THE FIT FORMULA AND NUTRITION

Notice in the table how the FIT Formula applies to nutritional fitness. If you eat too little or too much of one or more nutrients, you are not eating a balanced diet. In time, eating too many or too few nutrients affects your health. In the same way, your health can be weakened by a steady diet of "junk food," fad diets, fast foods, and incorrect use of vitamin and mineral supplements.

Fitness Target Zones and Nutrition

Consume the recommended number of servings from each of the four food groups.

Frequency	Eat three meals a day. An occasional snack is allowed.
Intensity	The number of Calories you consume each day should fall within the range recommended for your sex and age group.
Time	Eat meals at regular intervals, such as morning, noon, and evening.

When selecting foods, determine your own particular nutritional requirements. All people need the same nutrients, but they do not necessarily need the same amounts of each. As the U.S. RDA shows, a person's nutrient needs vary according to age, sex, height, and weight. Young people who are going through puberty and those who are still growing have special nutritional needs. They should eat foods high in potassium, calcium, and iron. These minerals aid in the development of bones and blood. By eating the correct number of servings from the four food groups, including foods high in calcium, potassium, and iron, you probably are consuming a balanced diet.

EATING DISORDERS

While poor nutrition can contribute to some health problems, eating disorders can also be harmful to your health. Two of the most common eating disorders are anorexia nervosa and bulimia. Both disorders occur most often among teenagers and young adults and more often among girls and women than boys and men.

ANOREXIA NERVOSA *Anorexia nervosa* is an eating disorder in which an individual severely limits food intake. People with this problem consider themselves overweight, even if they are dangerously underweight. To become thinner, anorexics suppress their bodies' normal urges to eat. Some anorexics exercise excessively to lose weight. Anorexics have been known to lose up to 50 percent of their normal weight. Anorexia can cause vitamin and mineral deficiencies, severe malnutrition, and dangerous loss of body fluids. If left untreated, anorexia nervosa can result in severe health problems or even death.

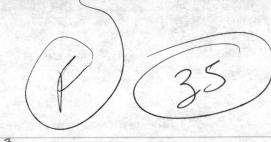

1. set, 10 or 15, little, lots (-1) ¹⁻³

2. how many reps you are going to do in one set
   (a set amount of reps then rest, and so on)

3. the number of times you are going to do it (-1)

4. something you do in a period of time. (-1)

5. 2 to 3 days week

6. it causes overload (-1)

7. 10 to 15

8. 10 to 15 5-10 (-1)

9. it loosens up the muscles, and it helps
   you get ready to workout.

10. (-4)

11. it helps your stamina (-1t)

12. deeply and when you are using your most
    strength (-1)

13. (-1)

14. (-3)

15. overload principle is when you lift to much and
    it hinders your training because you can
    hurt yourself. (-2)

16. T (-1)

17. T (18½)

18. 8

19. 4

20. B⁺

21. B — become more flexible & to gain more
22. B not shown

Matching

1. e
2. a
3. b
4. q
5. m
6. k
7. l i
8. o

9. n
10. p
11. g
12. h
13. g
14. d
15. d
16. f

a
b
c
d
e
f
g
k
l

j
x
v
n
n
p
p
q

BULIMIA People with *bulimia* show a pattern of overeating followed by forced vomiting or use of laxatives to rid the body of food. Bulimia differs from anorexia nervosa in that a bulimic's weight might be normal. This disorder can contribute to kidney failure, urinary tract infections, ulcers, and other serious health problems.

Anorexics and bulimics often try to hide what they are doing, deny it, or are reluctant to accept help. If someone you know shows symptoms of these diseases, you might talk to them about your concerns and encourage them to seek professional help.

MAKING NUTRITIOUS FOOD CHOICES

While many of your meals might be selected and prepared by other people, most teenagers make their own food choices for breakfast and lunch. These guidelines can help you make nutritious food choices:

● **Eat a variety of foods.** Choose not only from each food group, but from within each of the groups.

● **Try to reach your target weight and to maintain it.** Be aware of the number of Calories that you eat.

● **Avoid too much fat, especially saturated fat.** Choose lean meat, fish, poultry, dried beans and peas, low fat or skim milk. Limit your intake of fried foods.

● **Eat complex carbohydrates and ample fiber.** Choose starchy vegetables, fruits, and whole-grain breads and cereals. If possible, eat more raw than cooked or processed fruits and vegetables.

● **Avoid too much sugar.** Limit desserts to low-sugar, high nutrient choices, such as low-fat ice cream or ice milk, fresh fruit, and juices.

● **Limit your intake of salt.** Table salt contains sodium and chloride, two minerals your body needs in small amounts.

● **Eat three, regularly-spaced meals per day.** Do not skip breakfast. A snack is fine, provided it is nutritious and it does not cut down on your appetite for your evening meal.

● **Read the labels on food containers.** Labels list all ingredients in order of decreasing weight. A product called "Orange Drink" might have a label that reads, "filtered water, sugar, corn syrup, fumaric and citric acid (for tart flavor), ascorbic acid, artificial colors." By weight, this product contains more water than any other ingredient.

● **Drink plenty of water.** Drink about 2 quarts (eight 8-ounce glasses) of fluids per day. Fluids include water, milk, juice, and other beverages. People who lack the normal amount of body fluids are said to be *dehydrated.* As a result of dehydration, their bodies cannot function normally. When they replenish lost fluids by drinking liquids, they are said to be *rehydrated.* You can become seriously dehydrated if you are doing strenuous exercise in hot weather. In addition, dehydration can occur if you have an illness, such as stomach or intestinal flu, in which you lose a great deal of liquid.

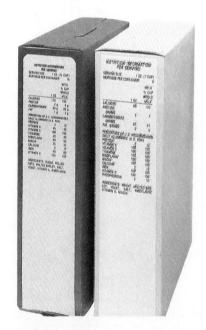

Read the labels on food containers.

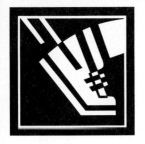

ACTIVITY

ANALYZING YOUR DIET

WORKSHEET 12-2

Use worksheet 12-2 to record the food you eat and analyze your eating habits.

Use this activity to record only what you normally eat to find out whether you need to make some changes. Use your worksheet to keep track of all foods and beverages you consume for three days. Write down each food and the portion size. Include gravies, sauces, spreads, and snacks. At the end of the three days, follow the directions on the worksheet to analyze your eating habits and total your score. Check your rating on the chart and record it on your worksheet.

Rating Chart: Analyzing Your Diet

Rating	Score
Very Good	14–15
Good	12–13
Fair	10–11
Low	9 or less

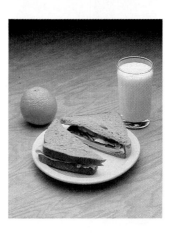

Choose a small meal before exercising.

EATING BEFORE EXERCISING

Some athletes mistakenly think that they need a steak, a "high energy" drink, or a food supplement before they compete or exercise. Steak is high in protein and fat, both of which are digested slowly. As a result, steak eaten within two hours of the activity might interfere with a person's performance. Similarly, scientists have found that drinking a beverage high in sugar before or during exercise actually can decrease the level of performance. Athletes do *not* need to drink so-called "sports drinks" unless a medical doctor advises it. Use the guidelines below to determine what to eat or drink before exercising.

● **Eat 1 to 3 hours before exercising.** The time you eat before exercising depends on your choice of food and the amount of time it takes your body to digest the food.

● **Eat what you like as long as it does not disagree with you.** Most athletes eat less protein and fat, and more complex carbohydrates.

● **Eat a small, easily digested meal.** You might choose a meal such as the one shown here. If you are really nervous before competition, you might try a liquid meal of about 900 calories in 16 ounces of liquid. However, limit your consumption of all-liquid meals.

● **Avoid snacks before and during exercise and competition.** You may snack during an activity if the activity lasts more than 90 minutes. Your body does not have enough time to digest a snack eaten during a short activity.

● **Drink fluids before, during, and after competition.** Drink water rather than special sport drinks.

CHAPTER REVIEW

MULTIPLE CHOICE

Choose the letter of the best answer.

1. Fruits, molasses, sugar, and honey contain (a) simple carbohydrates. (b) complex carbohydrates. (c) fiber. (d) protein.

2. Foods that contain a high ratio of nutrients to Calories are considered (a) empty Calories. (b) complete proteins. (c) incomplete proteins. (d) nutritionally dense.

3. Which nutrient provides twice as much energy per gram as carbohydrates? (a) protein (b) minerals (c) vitamins (d) fats

4. Which substance is not digestible? (a) fiber (b) complex carbohydrates (c) minerals (d) fats

5. Which is a source of incomplete protein? (a) fruit (b) milk (c) molasses (d) beans

6. Which product contains unsaturated fat? (a) bacon (b) lard (c) corn oil (d) butter

7. How many of the 22 amino acids does your body manufacture in your cells? (a) 4 (b) 6 (c) 8 (d) 14

8. Which vitamin dissolves in water, but does not dissolve in fat? (a) A (b) B (c) D (d) K

9. Which nutrient helps carry wastes out of and nutrients into your cells? (a) vitamins (b) minerals (c) fats (d) water

10. From which food group do you need only two servings per day? (a) meat-poultry-fish-beans (b) bread-cereal (c) fruit-vegetable (d) milk

MATCHING

Match the definition in Column I with the term it defines in Column II.

Column I

11. method of classifying foods
12. classified as saturated or unsaturated
13. water-soluble or fat-soluble
14. made of amino acid units
15. foods with all 8 essential amino acids
16. nutients that provide energy
17. waxy, fat-like substance
18. study of foods and how they nourish the body
19. type of carbohydrate your body cannot digest
20. food substances needed for cell growth and maintenance

Column II

a. carbohydrates
b. cholesterol
c. complete proteins
d. fats
e. fiber
f. four food groups
g. nutrients
h. nutrition
i. protein
j. vitamins

FOCUS ON FITNESS

CONTINUOUS RHYTHMICAL EXERCISES

Dr. T. K. Cureton pioneered the continuous rhythmical exercise program at the University of Illinois. The program includes calisthenics, jogging, and other slow-moving activities. Your goal is to keep your heart rate elevated during the entire exercise program by continually moving. Between exercises, you jog or slowly run in place. The sample program shown here lasts about 10 minutes. You can lengthen it by repeating the cycle of exercises.

CONTINUOUS RHYTHMICAL EXERCISE

Exercise	Length of Time or Number of Repetitions
Walk briskly in a circle	30 seconds
Jog in a circle	60 seconds
Side Stretcher	5 to each side
Lateral Shuffle (circle left)	30 seconds
Standing Heel Touch	10
Lateral Shuffle (circle right)	30 seconds
Trunk Curl	5
Jog in a circle	30 seconds
Side Leg Lift	5 to each side
Long Stride Step in circle	30 seconds
Partner Pull-Up	5
Skip in circle	30 seconds
Knee Dip	5 with each leg
Jog in a circle	60 seconds
Walk briskly in a circle	60 seconds

SIDE STRETCHER

● See page 10 for directions for this exercise.

KNEE DIP

1. Stand facing a partner. Hold each other's right hand as if shaking hands.
2. Stand on right foot and squat down. Your partner remains standing. Squat until your right knee is bent at a 90° angle. Your left leg is straight.
3. Use your partner's hand only for balance. Use your left arm and your partner's hand to lift yourself only if you cannot lift yourself without help.
4. Change legs and hands and repeat.

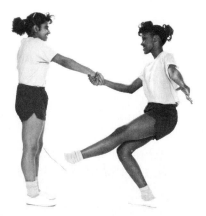

STRIDE STEP

• See page 21 for directions for this exercise.

PARTNER PULL-UP

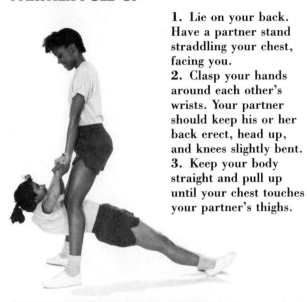

1. Lie on your back. Have a partner stand straddling your chest, facing you.
2. Clasp your hands around each other's wrists. Your partner should keep his or her back erect, head up, and knees slightly bent.
3. Keep your body straight and pull up until your chest touches your partner's thighs.

TRUNK CURL (ARMS EXTENDED)

1. Lie on your back with your arms extended to your sides. Bend your knees at a 90° angle.
2. Roll your head and shoulders forward and upward. Roll up until your shoulder blades leave the floor. *Caution:* Do not lift your back off the floor.
3. Return to starting position and repeat.

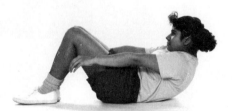

SIDE LEG RAISE

• See page 98 for directions for this exercise.

LATERAL SHUFFLE

1. Stand with your feet apart.
2. Move your left foot sideways, and then pull your right foot up to it. Continue to move your left foot and pull your right foot to it.
3. Repeat, moving your right foot sideways, and then pulling your left foot up to it.

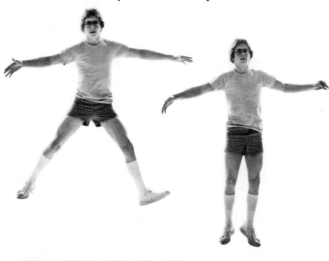

STANDING HEEL TOUCH

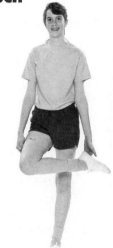

1. Stand and lift your right leg, bending knee. Turn your leg outward so your knee points out and heel points in.
2. Reach down with your left hand and touch your right heel.
3. Return to starting position and repeat using right hand to touch left heel.

VARYING THE PROGRAM Vary the exercise program these ways:
• Alternate exercises from Chapters 6 through 10.
• Be sure to include exercises for all parts of fitness.
• Alternate calisthenics with walking, jogging, skipping, lateral shuffle, or other movements.
• Form a large circle when doing this program as a group.

13

LIVING WITH STRESS

CHAPTER OBJECTIVES

After reading this chapter, you should be able to:

✔ Define the term "stress" and list causes of stress.

✔ Discuss the emotional and physical effects of stress.

✔ Discuss how to manage stress in everyday life.

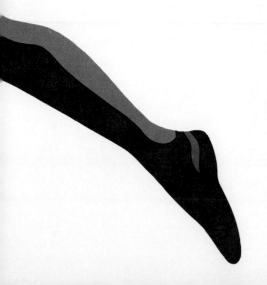

Hundreds of years ago, human beings lived quite differently than we do today. They had to hunt wild animals for food and to protect themselves. Sometimes people had to flee for safety. They used the "fight or flight" response—or stress response—to survive. The *stress response* is your body's way of preparing you to adapt to demanding situations. If danger presents itself, your stress response prepares your body for great bursts of energy, which can be used to either face the danger or avoid it. For example, if a bear were running toward you, your heart rate would increase, your muscles would tense, and your body would produce certain chemicals to help you run away. Of course, encountering a bear is an unusual situation. This chapter will discuss how stress affects you, and what you can do to manage stress in your daily life, even if you never have to flee from a bear.

WHAT IS STRESS?

Stress is the body's reaction to a demanding situation. A series of physical changes takes place automatically when you are in a highly stressful situation. Special glands send a chemical called adrenaline into your blood, the pupils of your eyes enlarge, and your body temperature rises. These and other physical changes prepare your body to deal with the demanding situation.

What causes stress? Basically, anything that causes you to worry or get excited, or causes other emotional and physical changes will cause stress. Something that causes or contributes to stress is called a *stressor*. For adults, stressors might include bills, vacation plans, responsibilities at work, and family conflicts. Common stressors for teenagers might be certain assignments in school, grades, sporting events, family arguments, and peer pressures. Each situation is a stressor that causes changes in the body's normal functioning.

EUSTRESS AND DISTRESS

While stressful situations affect the body's functioning, not all stressful experiences are considered harmful. Scientists use the term *eustress* to describe "good stress." Situations that might produce eustress include riding a roller coaster, successfully completing a gymnastic routine, passing a driving test, meeting new people, and playing in the school band. Eustress helps enrich your life and make it more enjoyable by helping you meet challenges and do your best.

On the other hand, unpleasant situations can also cause stress. The word *distress* is sometimes used to describe "bad stress." Situations that cause worrying, sorrow, anger, or physical pain would certainly produce distress.

Obviously, a situation that causes eustress for one person can be distressful for another. For example, an outgoing person might look forward to joining extracurricular activities at school; a shy person might dread it. Also, a similar situation can be eustressful or distressful for the same person at different times. For example, if you have prepared for a test, taking that test might cause eustress. Another test that you have not prepared for might cause distress.

Ideally, you should strive for the right amount of stress—neither too much nor too little. These pictures illustrate this idea. Too much stress can cause you to "burn out," possibly leading to emotional and physical problems. On the other hand, avoiding stress altogether would deprive you of the opportunity to live a full and productive life. In fact, small amounts of stress help you prepare for greater stressful situations in the future. For example, exercise can be considered a stressor, but regular exercise makes you fit, healthy, and better able to handle future stressful situations.

HAVE YOU HEARD?

The prefix "eu" in "eustress" is taken from "euphoria," meaning a feeling of well-being.

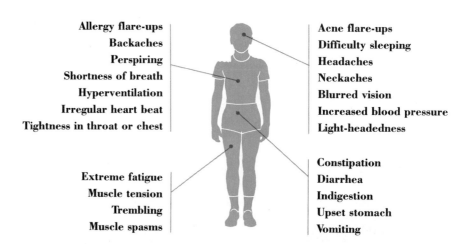

Allergy flare-ups
Backaches
Perspiring
Shortness of breath
Hyperventilation
Irregular heart beat
Tightness in throat or chest

Acne flare-ups
Difficulty sleeping
Headaches
Neckaches
Blurred vision
Increased blood pressure
Light-headedness

Extreme fatigue
Muscle tension
Trembling
Muscle spasms

Constipation
Diarrhea
Indigestion
Upset stomach
Vomiting

Effects of stress on the body

CAUSES OF DISTRESS

In order to control the amount of stress in your life, you must be clear about the cause of the stress. Because the kind of stressors that affect your total fitness most is the distress type, this section takes a more detailed look at the causes of distress.

PHYSICAL STRESSORS Conditions of your body and the environment that directly affect your physical well-being can be categorized as physical stressors. Examples include thirst, hunger, overexposure to heat or cold, lack of sleep, excessive physical exercise, illness, weather extremes, pollution, noise, accidents, and catastrophes such as floods, storms, and fires. People who are fit and healthy are much more able to adapt to the changes or stresses produced by physical stressors.

EMOTIONAL STRESSORS Emotions such as worry, fear, anger, grief, and depression are powerful stressors. Each of these emotions usually stems from or leads to another stressor. For example, you worry about something or you are afraid of something. The "something" is as much a stressor as the emotion it produces.

SOCIAL STRESSORS Social stressors arise from your relationships with other people. Each day you experience situations that involve your family members, friends, teachers, and others. Think about what stressors might stem from the social situations in your life.

As a teenager, you are exposed to many social stressors. In fact, most of the significant stress you experience probably is caused by social stressors. This makes sense in light of all the changes and preparations for change that are part of the teen years. The chart on page 166 lists some of the stressors you might encounter as a teenager.

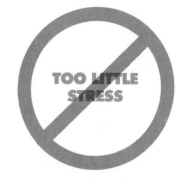

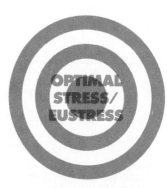

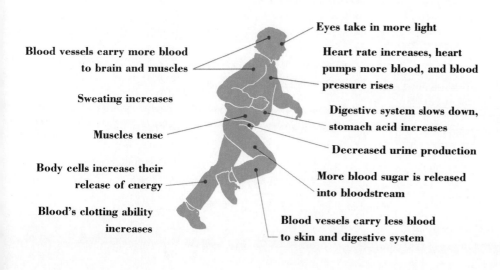

Eyes take in more light

Heart rate increases, heart pumps more blood, and blood pressure rises

Blood vessels carry more blood to brain and muscles

Sweating increases

Digestive system slows down, stomach acid increases

Muscles tense

Decreased urine production

Body cells increase their release of energy

More blood sugar is released into bloodstream

Blood's clotting ability increases

Blood vessels carry less blood to skin and digestive system

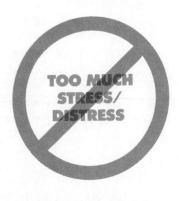

Some amount of stress in life is good.

EFFECTS OF STRESS

As you know, physical changes caused by stress prepare your body to deal with demanding situations. Even while under stress, you are probably not aware that many of them occur. These changes, however, lead to other reactions that you might have noticed.

Have you ever experienced extreme fatigue, light-headedness, or upset stomach due to stress? These and other reactions are common physical reactions to stressors. Of course, these reactions vary from one person to another. They usually last only a short period of time, disappearing once the source of the stress is removed. However, high levels of stress and prolonged periods of stress can lead to many conditions. For example, the increased stomach acid caused by stress can lead to ulcers. High blood pressure caused by stress can lead to cardiovascular problems, such as stroke. Prolonged stress also can lower the effectiveness of the body's immune system, making a person more susceptible to disease. While the precise role of stress in causing diseases is a debated topic, some doctors think that more than half of the health problems in the United States requiring medical attention are stress related. The motivation to deal effectively with one's stress, especially distress, is clear.

Use worksheet 13-1 to find out how prone you are to stress. If you are prone to stress, consider using the procedures for managing stress described in this chapter.

WORKSHEET 13-1

Use worksheet 13-1 to determine how prone you are to stress.

Common Emotional Reactions to Stressors

- Feeling upset or nervous
- Anger, anxiety, fear
- Criticizing others
- Forgetfulness
- Frustration
- Difficulty making decisions
- Difficulty paying attention
- Feeling hassled or hurried
- Irritability
- Lack of motivation
- Mild depression
- Not being able to enjoy yourself
- Overeating or loss of appetite
- Withdrawal or boredom
- Substance abuse

Common Sources of Teenage Stress

- Poor grades
- Family conflicts
- Death in the family
- Move to another city
- Serious family illness
- Feelings of loneliness
- Substance abuse
- Poor eating habits
- Lack of exercise
- Delaying school assignments
- Taking tests
- Change or loss of friends, boyfriend, or girlfriend
- Trouble with school or legal authorities

Diseases Thought to be Stress-Related

- Allergies
- Arthritis
- Asthma
- Backaches
- Cancer
- Cardiovascular diseases
- Colds
- Diabetes
- Flu
- Hay fever
- Infections
- Migraine headaches
- Ulcers

MANAGING STRESS

By now you might feel a bit overwhelmed by the many causes of distress and their effects on your physical and emotional well-being. But you probably already deal effectively with most distress every day. Distress in your daily life is unavoidable; it is a part of life and always has been. However, the sources of stress might change over time and from place to place. For example, diseases such as smallpox and polio used to be sources of distress, not only from the diseases themselves but from fear of the diseases. Thanks to medical advancements, these sources of distress have been largely eliminated. However, air and noise pollution, crowded conditions, and other aspects of modern life are sources of stress our ancestors generally did not have to deal with.

Fortunately, you can take steps to manage the stress in your life. When a problem or situation seems distressful, try one or more of the suggestions given below and on the next three pages. Some might seem simple and obvious, but they work.

● **Rest in a quiet place.** Sit or lie down indoors or outdoors.

● **Reduce breathing rate.** Sit or lie quietly. Take several long, slow breaths in through your nose and out through your mouth.

● **Reduce mental activity.** Sometimes, it is best to get rid of the thoughts that cause distress until you can deal with them more effectively. Counting as you breathe slowly is one way to do this. You might also try imagining something pleasant and peaceful, such as a favorite outdoor scene. Listening to music or watching television might also provide an appropriate diversion.

● **Reduce muscle tension.** Relaxing your muscles to reduce muscle tension is an effective way to help reduce distress. When you feel tense, contract some of your muscles, such as those in your arms, and then suddenly release the contraction, letting your arms go limp. Try this technique for all your muscles.

● **Use exercise as a diversion.** An excellent way to relieve distress is through physical activity. Exercise helps reduce stress by relaxing tense muscles and burning extra fuel and fat in your blood. You might try the exercises described in the activity on page 170 in addition to sports or other exercise you might enjoy.

● **Identify the cause of the stress.** When you are ready to deal with the stressor, first identify it clearly. For example, anger might be causing you stress, but try to identify what is making you angry.

● **Tackle one thing at a time.** Sometimes several problems pile up. Ask yourself, "Which problems can I do something about now?" "Which can wait a while?" "Which problems cannot be changed?"

● **Take action.** Rather than worrying about a problem, do what you can to solve it. This involves making decisions and carrying them out. When making a decision, it is important to look at several choices, consider the results of each, and choose the best.

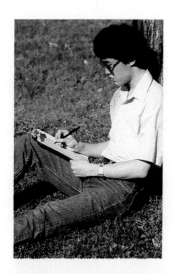

Relaxing in a quiet place can reduce stress.

- **Manage time effectively.** Between school work, extracurricular activities, part-time jobs, friendships, and family obligations, the life of a teenager can be hectic. Prioritize your activities so that you have time for the most important things. Learn to say "no" to new responsibilities or activities if you cannot give them the time required.

- **Accept what cannot be changed.** Not all problems can be solved the way you would like them to be, but they can still be dealt with effectively to reduce stress. You might try to change your feelings toward the situation by looking at the bright side and turning something negative into something positive. For example, suppose you were feeling stress from guilt or shame about something you did. The past cannot be changed, but you can deal with the stress by first admitting that you are human and are going to make mistakes, by taking action to correct the situation, and by avoiding that situation in the future.

- **Think positively.** When you think negatively, you are more likely to make mistakes and feel distressed. Thinking positive thoughts might help reduce or eliminate distress. For example, by thinking that you will get a hit in a softball game instead of worrying about striking out will help relieve stress.

- **Change the way you perceive a stressor.** A poet once remarked, "When I see conflict, I see opportunity for understanding." Similarly, you can perceive a stressor in terms of a problem or in terms of a solution. Perception also affects how you interpret people's actions. For example, you might interpret a friend's silence as anger when it might not be that at all.

- **Do not mask your problems.** Sometimes people who are experiencing distress mask the problem or try to avoid it. They might try to "hide behind" alcohol or drugs. In the long run, masking or hiding the problem usually leads to more, not less, distress, and the original problem remains.

- **Try not to let the little things bother you.** Many things in life create stress, but many of them simply are not worth it. For example, the anger you might feel at a brother or sister who wore one of your shirts is easily controllable and probably not worth the stress that your anger puts on you or your family.

- **Be willing to make adjustments.** The expression, "A branch that is able to bend will not break," applies to people as well as trees. People who learn to bend a little, or who are able to adjust from time to time, can handle distress better than people who cannot adjust.

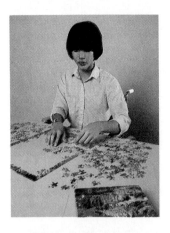

Take a break from a stressful situation.

STRESS MANAGEMENT, FITNESS, AND GOOD HEALTH

The guidelines listed here can also help you manage stress:

● **Eat a nutritious, well-balanced diet.** Poor nutrition can contribute to health problems, which in turn makes it harder for you to deal with distress. Chapter 12 discusses the importance of good nutrition.

● **Avoid unnecessary, distressful situations.** If you know a situation will be stressful, and there is no reason to experience the distress, you can usually avoid it. For example, if you choose not to drink alcohol and you are invited to a party where it will be served, it might be best not to attend.

● **Get enough sleep.** Lack of sleep can contribute to distress. In fact, lack of sleep for long periods of time is itself a stressor. Problems that seem very large to a fatigued person might be easily handled by a person who is well rested. Try to get at least 8 hours of sleep per day.

● **Pay attention to your body.** With practice, you can learn to recognize the physical signs of stress listed on page 166. Pay attention to how your body reacts in different situations. Muscle tension and increased heart rate are both signs of stress. If you experience physical signs of distress, use some of the stress-management techniques described in this chapter.

● **Have fun.** Laughter can help lessen distress. Take time in your schedule to laugh and have fun. Let yourself enjoy life.

GETTING HELP

Often people need help in managing their stress. Parents, family members, teachers, members of the clergy, and friends can be sources of help and support. School counselors, school nurses, physicians, and other specially trained people can provide advice about stress management. In addition, many communities have health professionals to help people manage stress. A doctor, school counselor, referral service in a hospital, or the yellow pages of your local telephone book can direct you to sources of help in your community.

HAVE YOU HEARD?

Biofeedback is one way to change your body's reaction to stress. In biofeedback, you use a machine or other method to monitor your heart rate, breathing rate, muscle tension, or some other body reaction. A biofeedback specialist helps you try to change your body's reactions, using the feedback from the machine.

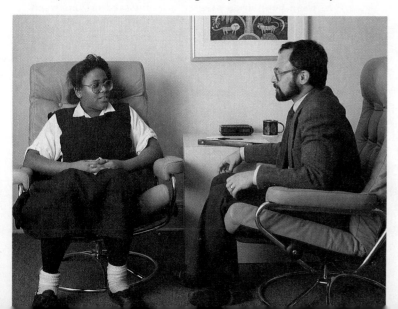

Get help when you need it.

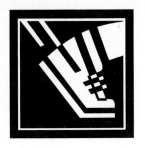

ACTIVITY

MEASURING AND RESPONDING TO STRESS

WORKSHEET 13-2
Use worksheet 13-2 to measure your own stress and how you respond to it.

Use worksheet 13-2 to get an idea of the amount of distress in your life. Find your score on the worksheet chart. If you have a high score, consider using some of the stress-management methods discussed in this chapter, including these exercises.

ELEPHANT SWING

1. Stand with your feet apart. Bend at your waist and let your arms hang in front of you.
2. Swing your arms and upper body from side to side. You may lift your heels off the floor for balance, if needed. Keep your neck and trunk muscles relaxed.

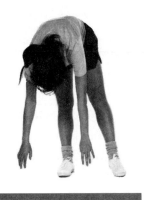

NECK ROLL

1. Sit with your legs crossed and eyes closed.
2. Slowly roll your head in a half circle to the left. Then slowly roll your head in a half circle to the right. *Caution:* Do not roll your head in a full circle or tip your head backward.

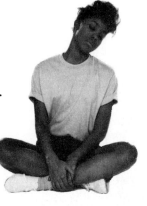

PEN DROP

1. Sit in a chair with a pen or pencil in your hand. Slouch forward. Close your eyes and let your head hang down.
2. Tighten your leg muscles, and then relax them. Breathe slowly.
3. Continue to breathe slowly until you hear the pen hit the floor when it drops from your hand.

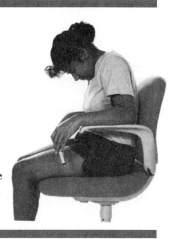

BODY BOARD

1. Lie on your side. Hold your arms over your head.
2. Stiffen your body as if you were a wooden board. Then relax your muscles.

3. Let your body roll forward or backward. Continue to relax your muscles.

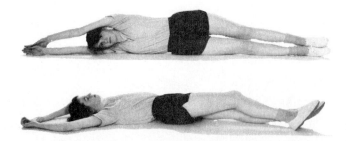

CHAPTER REVIEW

MULTIPLE CHOICE
Choose the letter of the best answer.

1. To reduce respiration during periods of stress, try (a) exercising vigorously. (b) sitting quietly and breathing deeply. (c) going indoors. (d) counting to ten.

2. Which would probably not cause you stress? (a) a serious illness in the family (b) getting ready to go on a school trip (c) going to a class well-prepared (d) the first day of a new job

3. Ideally, you should try to have (a) no stress in your life. (b) only distress. (c) the right amount of stress, concentrating on eustress. (d) as much distress as possible.

4. Which is an example of a physical stressor? (a) anger (b) fear (c) worry (d) lack of sleep

5. Social stressors arise from (a) pollution. (b) relationships with other people. (c) illness. (d) too much exercise.

6. During stress, your (a) blood pressure rises. (b) heart pumps less blood. (c) digestive system speeds up. (d) heart rate decreases.

7. During stress, (a) sweating decreases. (b) muscles relax. (c) stomach acid increases. (d) blood does not clot.

8. What physical changes occur in the body in a stressful situation? (a) Some physical changes occur. (b) No physical changes occur. (c) You have complete control over all physical changes. (d) The "fight or flight response" does not occur.

9. A person will be better able to manage stress if he or she (a) ignores problems. (b) is unwilling to make adjustments in life. (c) tries to handle all problems at once. (d) thinks positively.

10. How many hours of sleep each night should you get? (a) 6 (b) 7 (c) 8 (d) 11

MATCHING
Match the definition in Column I with the term it defines in Column II.

Column I	Column II
11. the body's reaction to a demanding situation	a. distress
12. fight or flight response	b. eustress
13. reactions of worry, sorrow, anger, pain, and other undesirable reactions	c. stress
14. something that causes or contributes to stress	d. stressor
15. "good" stress	e. stress response

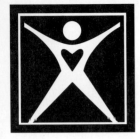

FOCUS ON FITNESS

FRISBEE® GOLF

Frisbee golf is a relatively new sport that can be played by people of all ages. It is not an especially good activity for building health-related fitness, but it can be a great way to relax and reduce stress. Above all, Frisbee golf is just fun if you play for enjoyment rather than competition.

As the name suggests, the game is played like golf. Eighteen "holes" or goals are arranged throughout the course. The object of the game is to throw the Frisbee from each "tee" into each goal with the least possible throws. Each hole has a "par" of the recommended number of throws to get the Frisbee in the goal. You should try to achieve par or less for each hole. Your score is the total number of throws for 18 holes of Frisbee golf.

More and more communities have special Frisbee golf courses located in parks. However, you can also design your own course. You might use rope, hula hoops, waste baskets, or chalk lines on the ground as the holes or goals. Simply arrange them around a large area. If space is limited you might have fewer than 18 holes and repeat the holes until you have played 18.

If you are playing for fun and relaxation, it is best not to be too competitive. You might want to compare your score to par and try to improve rather than comparing your score to someone else's.

To increase the fitness gained from the activity, consider doing exercises at each hole. The sample course on the next page gives you some examples of exercises you might do at each hole for a 9-hole course. The exercises can vary, but the first and last holes should include warm-up and cool-down exercises respectively.

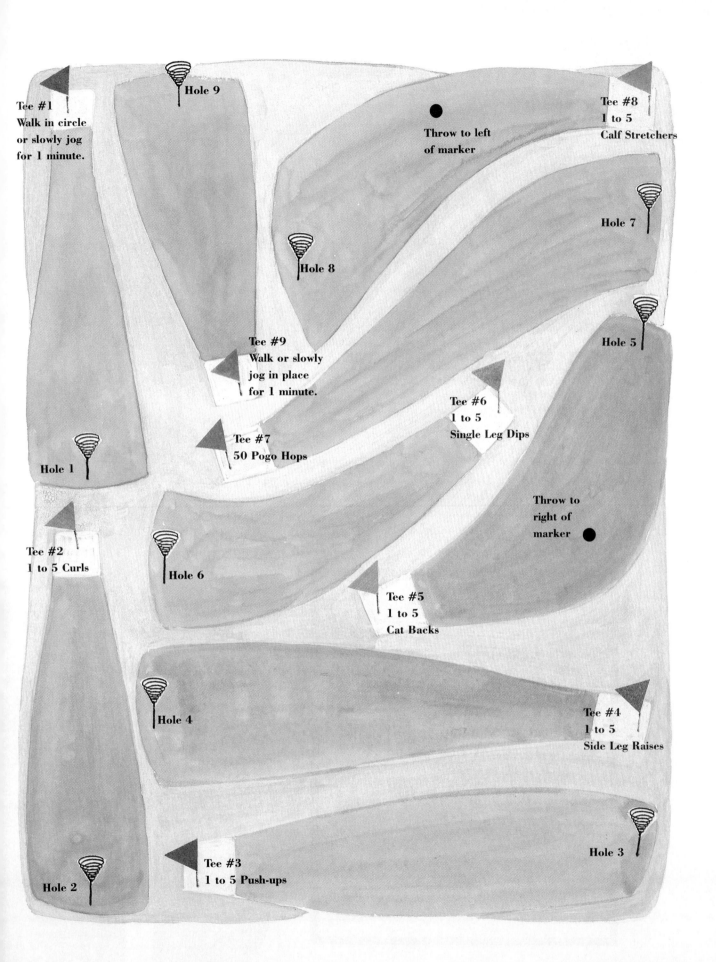

Tee #1
Walk in circle
or slowly jog
for 1 minute.

Hole 9

Throw to left
of marker

Tee #8
1 to 5
Calf Stretchers

Hole 7

Hole 8

Hole 5

Tee #9
Walk or slowly
jog in place
for 1 minute.

Tee #6
1 to 5
Single Leg Dips

Tee #7
50 Pogo Hops

Hole 1

Throw to
right of
marker

Tee #2
1 to 5 Curls

Hole 6

Tee #5
1 to 5
Cat Backs

Tee #4
1 to 5
Side Leg Raises

Hole 4

Hole 3

Tee #3
1 to 5 Push-ups

Hole 2

14

MAKING CONSUMER CHOICES

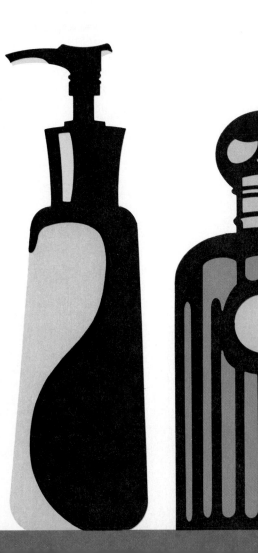

CHAPTER OBJECTIVES

After reading this chapter, you should be able to:

✔ Discuss the importance of being an informed health consumer.

✔ Name reliable sources of health- and fitness-related information.

✔ Evaluate health- and fitness-related information.

✔ Describe your responsiblities as a health consumer.

✔ Name and describe examples of health- and fitness-related misconceptions and quackery.

Have you noticed how advertising for health and fitness products has increased during the past several years? People are bombarded by newspaper, magazine, television, and radio advertisements for these products. Many entertainers and athletes have endorsed health items. But is a product effective simply because it is widely advertised or endorsed? This chapter discusses some steps that can help you become a wise consumer—or purchaser—of health and fitness products.

WHAT IS QUACKERY?

Some people are in a hurry to lose body fat or gain muscular strength. They get impatient or discouraged with gradual improvements. Often, people who want quick results are those who are persuaded to buy useless health or fitness products and services. Such people are likely to become victims of quackery. *Quackery* is a method of advertising or selling that uses false claims to lure people into buying products that are worthless, or even harmful.

If you have questions about health or fitness, ask an expert's advice. A number of people are qualified to give reliable, accurate advice. Talk to a medical doctor (M.D.), a registered nurse (R.N.), or a health education teacher. A physical educator or physical therapist is qualified to advise you about exercise and fitness. A *registered dietitian (R.D.)* is qualified to advise you about diet and food.

Avoid consulting a nutritionist. The title "nutritionist" does not necessarily mean that a person is educated or trained in nutrition. Many states require no specialized training for this title and anyone can be called nutritionist. Similarly, staff members in health clubs are usually not required to have specialized training in physical fitness. Neither nutritionists nor health club staff employees are considered reliable sources of health or fitness information unless they have the credentials described above.

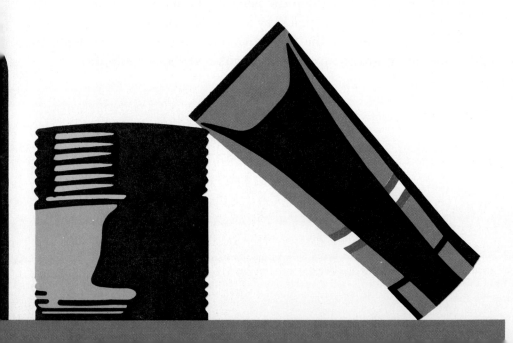

WORKSHEET 14-1

Use worksheet 14-1 to find out how much you know about quackery.

HAVE YOU HEARD?

By law, labels on food products must show the ingredients listed in order of decreasing amounts. However, the law does not require manufacturers to indicate the *exact amount* of each ingredient in a product.

DETECTING QUACKERY

Frequently, you can spot health or fitness quackery by identifying sales techniques or tricks such as the ones listed below:

● **False credentials** A quack might claim to be a doctor or to have degrees from colleges and universities. However, the degree might be in a subject totally unrelated to health and physical fitness. It might come from an unaccredited school, or it might be a fake. You can verify credentials by checking with your local or state health authorities or professional organizations.

● **Immediate results** Be suspicious if the salesperson promises immediate, effortless, or guaranteed results.

● **Sales pitch** Look for words and phrases such as, "miracle," "secret remedy," "breakthrough," and "clinical studies show that...." A health quack is likely to use these and similar terms in a sales pitch.

● **Mail-order sales** Be cautious of mail-order offers and money-back guarantees. You cannot examine mail-order products before buying them. A guarantee is only as good as the company that backs it.

● **Lack of medical support** Some quacks claim that the American Medical Association (or other groups) is against them only because the organization itself will not profit from the sale of the product.

● **Brand new (untested) products** Quacks do not subject their products to a thorough scientific testing. Usually, the product is rushed onto the market in order to make money as quickly as possible.

How knowledgeable are you about quackery? You can complete worksheet 14-1 to find out how knowledgeable you are about quackery.

HEALTH QUACKERY

Today, people are very concerned about nutrition, and most are willing to try a new health product. As a result, the market is flooded with health products, many of which are useless. Some products are not in themselves harmful. However, false advertising claims give people unrealistic expectations about the benefits these products can provide. You can spot nutritional quackery when advertisements claim that a product will do one of the following: increase muscle development, promote hair growth, cure acne, or make wrinkles disappear.

FOOD SUPPLEMENTS A *food supplement* is a product intended to add to a person's nutrient consumption. It is one type of health product that usually is unnecessary and sometimes is harmful. For example, health experts consider products such as amino-acid supplements and weight-control supplements a waste of money. Food supplements often are produced as syrups, powders, or tablets. Generally, they are sold in health-food stores or through the mail. In special cases, people do need to supplement their diets. For example, a doctor might prescribe supplements. In this case, use only the prescribed supplement.

FAD DIETS "Lose two pounds a day on the ice-cream diet!" "Rice diet works wonders!" "All-fruit diet dissolves fat!" How many of these and similar weight-loss claims have you heard? Each claim is false and is an example of a fad diet. Although *fad diets* are popular because they usually promise results in a short period of time, nearly all fad diets are nutritionally unbalanced. They often restrict eating to only one or two food groups, or even one specific food. For example, one weight-loss diet consists of eating only bananas and skim milk. Another fad diet calls for grapefruit before every meal. The digestion of grapefruit supposedly triggers reactions that result in fat loss. This diet sells a lot of grapefruit, but does not contribute to safe, steady weight loss.

FITNESS QUACKERY

People who are interested in physical fitness should be alert for fitness quackery. For instance, you probably have seen advertisements telling you that you can lose weight in one area of your body if you buy a certain device or machine for "spot reduction." Or, an unqualified fitness instructor might recommend spot exercises.

Spot exercises, which act only on one particular part of the body, do *not* remove fat. For example, doing trunk curls to remove excess fat at the waistline is not especially useful. When you do spot exercises, you might strengthen muscles in a particular place, but you are not "burning off" fat at that location.

To get rid of excess fat, you must use up more Calories than usual by doing cardiovascular endurance exercises. Note however, that exercise removes fat from all over your body—not just from one area. You cannot control the places from which fat is removed any more than you can control where fat accumulates when you eat too much.

HAVE YOU HEARD?

Advertisers often photograph models who are underweight to sell women's clothing. Advertisers want customers to think they will look as good as the models wearing the clothing. This practice promotes a very unrealistic standard. Very few people can be, or should be, as thin as these models.

The National Museum of Quackery in St. Louis, Missouri, has an exhibit of quack inventions from the past. Here, you can see many unusual gadgets. One invention is a machine that supposedly reduced the waistline by giving electric shocks. Another gadget is a belt that was claimed to be "a cure for any disease."

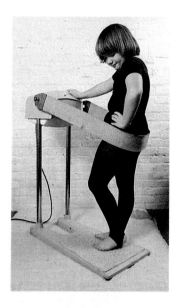

An ineffective exercise machine

INEFFECTIVE FITNESS PRODUCTS AND METHODS Some exercise programs are not effective for building fitness. Therefore, these programs are a waste of time. For example, *passive exercises* are not effective because they use machines or some other outside force to move your body instead of your own muscles. Most of the products described below provide a form of passive exercise:

● Rollers are machines that roll up and down your hips or legs. Quacks claim these machines roll off fat, just as the action of a rolling pin flattens dough. This claim is false. Rollers do not help remove fat.

● Vibrating machines, such as vibrating tables, belts, and pillows, are designed to shake body areas and "break up" fat cells. These devices do not remove fat, break up fat cells, or help a person lose weight.

● Motorized cycles, motorized rowing machines, and motorized tables move people while they are sitting or lying down. Motorized machines do not improve muscle strength because the people using the machines are not working their muscles on their own.

● Wearing a belt, shorts, or other type of tight garment does not reduce a person's waist or hip size, nor does it eliminate fat.

● Wrapping the entire body in cloths that have been soaked in a "magic" solution supposedly removes inches and eliminates fat. Wrapping the body in cloths does neither.

● Sauna baths, whirlpool baths, mineral baths, and steam baths might help a person feel clean. They might even make them feel very relaxed. However, these bath do not help a person lose fat, avoid colds or other diseases, or improve fitness. In fact, such baths can be harmful if a person stays in the bath too long and overheats. In addition, these baths can be dangerous if the person has a cardiovascular condition or is under the influence of alcohol or other drugs.

● A nonporous garment, such as a plastic sweat suit, is nearly airtight. As a result, wearing this clothing for active exercises raises the body's temperature and causes the wearer to perspire heavily. Some people claim that during this process their body fat melts and is eliminated through their skin pores. What they are really losing through their pores are body fluids—not fat. By wearing nonporous clothing, an exerciser risks both dehydration and overheating.

You already know that there is no quick, easy way to attain health or fitness goals. Both goals take planning and time to achieve. Similarly, there is no magic diet, product, or exercise program that will cause you to lose excess fat quickly, yet safely. Weight lost through a safe, steady program of reduced Calorie consumption and exercise is more likely to remain off than weight lost in a hurry.

Save your money and health by learning to recognize misconceptions. Education is the best safeguard against quackery.

EVALUATING BOOKS AND ARTICLES

Growing emphasis on health and fitness has led to the publication of thousands of books and articles on weight control and exercise. One study evaluated the accuracy of nutrition information published in 19 major magazines. Only five of the magazines published generally reliable information; eight others were sometimes reliable; the remaining six were unreliable. Thus, you should be aware that what you read about weight control and fitness could be misleading or incorrect.

Certain guidelines apply equally well to both weight-control and fitness literature. For instance, terms such as "secret formula," "melts fat," "tones muscles," "miraculous," or "quick" should not appear in the book or article. These terms are unscientific and are associated with health quackery sales techniques.

In additon, the author(s) should be an authority on the subject being presented. A newspaper or magazine writer is an acceptable author if this person accurately quotes a health specialist. The book should include the authors' qualifications. To prevent a conflict of interests, the author(s) should not be advertising or producing any health or fitness products. The guidelines below refer to both health literature and fitness literature. Use them to help you decide whether a book or an article is a reliable source of information.

Guidelines For Evaluating Books About Weight Control

● The author(s) or consultant(s) should be a registered dietition or an individual who has completed advanced study in nutrition.
● The book or article should contain information about a balanced diet and recommend exercises as well as a diet plan.
● Information should be included on how to cut down on Calories and fats by substituting one type of food for another.
● The diet plan should not favor one particular food or nutrient, nor should it decrease or omit any of the food groups or nutrients.
● A weight-loss plan should call for at least 1,000 to 1,200 Calories per day and no more than two pounds of weight loss per week.
● Methods for correcting bad nutritional habits should be provided.

Guidelines For Evaluating Books About Fitness

● The author(s) or consultant(s) should be a physical educator, physical therapist, or an individual who has completed advanced study in exercise physiology.
● Exercise discussions should include the principles of overload, progression, and specificity in addition to the FIT Formula.
● The recommended exercises should be safe and effective.
● The exercises should require the use of your own muscles. They should not be exercises that call for "effortless" devices.

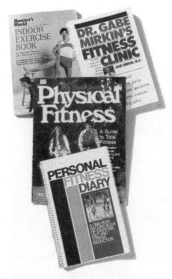

Fitness books and magazines have flooded the market.

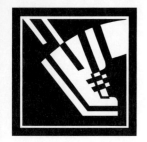

ACTIVITY

RECOGNIZING QUACKERY

WORKSHEET 14-2
Use Worksheet 14-2 to record your observations and comments.

Use this activity to evaluate an example of health, nutrition, or fitness quackery. Find an example in a book, magazine, or newspaper. Your example might be a story about how to get fit, lose weight, or lose inches. Or, your example might be an advertisement for a diet, food supplement, exercise program, exercise garment, or exercise machine. Follow these steps:

1. Make a photocopy of your example, or cut it out and paste it on a sheet of paper. Then write down the name of the publication where you found your example and the names and qualifications of the authors, if that information is given.

2. Review this chapter's information about health and fitness services and products. Then evaluate your example based on this information.

3. Record your observations and comments and answer the questions on worksheet 14-2.

4. If time permits, examine the other students' examples and evaluations. Decide whether or not you would buy the products in their examples and give reasons for your decisions.

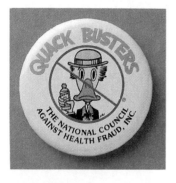

Organizations work to protect consumers from fraud.

RELIABLE CONSUMER ORGANIZATIONS

Many organizations work to protect consumers from misleading advertising and quackery. These organizations include the Federal Trade Commission, the Food and Drug Administration, the Consumer Product Safety Commission, the United States Postal Service, the Better Business Bureau, Consumers Union, the National Council Against Health Fraud, the American Medical Association, the American Dental Association, and the American College of Sports Medicine. These agencies receive and investigate consumer complaints and provide information to consumers.

As a consumer, you need to be informed about the products and services you use. Do not assume that every advertised product is safe and effective. While agencies such as the ones named above can provide information, you make the final decision about buying a product or service.

CHAPTER REVIEW

MULTIPLE CHOICE

Choose the letter of the best answer.

1. Which person is *least* qualified to answer questions about nutrition? (a) health education teacher (b) nurse (c) health club exercise instructor (d) registered dietician.

2. Which is most closely identified with health quackery? (a) well-tested product (b) medical endorsement (c) useful product (d) sales pitch

3. Which is *not* true of food supplements? (a) everyone needs them (b) sold in health food stores (c) sold by mail (d) often produced in powder, syrup, or tablet form

4. Which information might be found in an accurate weight-control article? (a) Calorie intake: 950 daily (b) weight loss: 4 pounds per week (c) 6 servings of fruits and vegetables, and 2 servings of milk products per day (d) food substitutions for reducing Calorie intake

5. Eating cereal for every meal for a month is an example of a (a) fad diet. (b) fitness program. (c) craving for certain nutrients. (d) child's diet.

6. Which is *least* likely to help you get rid of excess body fat? (a) cardiovascular endurance exercises (b) spot exercises (c) reduced Calorie diet (d) daily 30 minute walks

7. Which is *most* helpful for losing excess body fat? (a) cardiovascular endurance exercises (b) roller machines (c) motorized machines (d) sauna baths

8. Which does *not* occur when a person wearing a rubber suit is exercising vigorously? (a) loss of body fluid (b) higher body temperature (c) fat cells melt (d) heavy perspiration

9. Which is your best protection against health and fitness quackery? (a) money (b) education (c) luck (d) advertising

10. Which organization is *not* associated with consumer protection? (a) State Department (b) U.S. Postal Service (c) Better Business Bureau (d) Federal Trade Commission

MATCHING

Match the definition in Column I with the term it defines in Column II.

Column I

11. unnecessary health product
12. nutrition expert
13. using false claims to sell products
14. unbalanced diet
15. no contracting or stretching of muscles

Column II

a. fad diet
b. food supplement
c. passive exercises
d. quackery
e. registered dietician

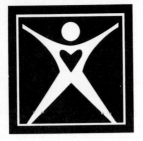

FOCUS ON FITNESS

INNER TUBE EXERCISES

You learned in Chapters 7 and 8 that overload is necessary to build strength and muscular endurance. Weight training and exercise machines are two ways to provide overload. These activities require special equipment that is usually quite expensive. Inner tube exercises provide an inexpensive and effective alternative to build strength and muscular endurance.

You will need a bicycle inner tube or a length of sturdy latex surgical tubing. If you are using an inner tube, wash the tube and then cut it on both sides of the valve stem. Tie the two ends of the tube together with a square knot. You might cut and tie more than one inner tube to use for different exercises. Long, thin tubes are easier to stretch than shorter, thicker tubes. You might start with a longer, thinner tube and work your way up to stretching a shorter, thicker tube.

As with any new activity, begin gradually. Start with the minimum number of repetitions and sets and gradually increase them. Follow the guidelines suggested in Chapters 7 and 8 as you exercise. As you improve, you might make a double loop with your tube or shorten the length of the tube to make the exercises more difficult.

ARM CURL

1. Loop the tube under your feet.
2. With your palms facing up, pull your hands to your chest. Keep your elbows against your sides.
3. Return to starting position. Complete 3 to 15 repetitions. Complete 1 to 3 sets.

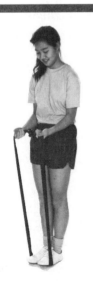

UPWARD ROW

1. Loop the tube under your feet.
2. Hold the tube with both hands, with your palms facing you. Gradually pull up on the tube, keeping your elbows high. Pull until your hands reach your chin.

3. Lower your hands to starting position. Complete 3 to 15 repetitions. Complete 1 to 3 sets.

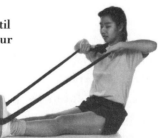

LEG SPREAD

1. Loop the tube around your feet.
2. Grasp the other end of the tube in your hands near your chest. Gradually spread your legs.

3. Return to starting position. Complete 3 to 15 repetitions. Complete 1 to 3 sets.

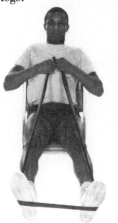 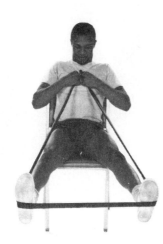

ONE-LEG PRESS

1. Loop the tube over one shoulder and under one foot.
2. Lift the foot that is on top of the tube. Gradually press. You might lean on a chair with one hand to help keep your balance.

3. Return to starting position. Complete 3 to 15 repetitions with each leg. Complete 1 to 3 sets.

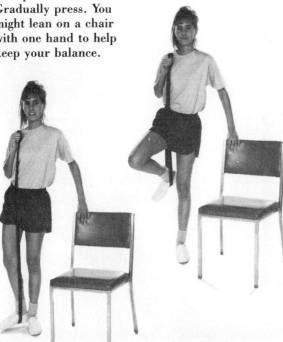

TOE PUSH

1. Loop the tube under your toes. Hold the other end with your hands.

2. Push with your feet by pointing your toes against the tube.
3. Return to starting position. Repeat 3 to 15 times. Complete 1 to 3 sets. You might hold the tube closer to your feet to make the exercise more difficult.

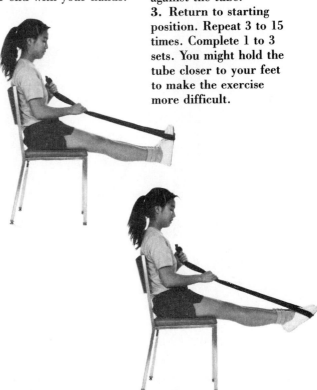

ARM DROP

1. Loop the tube over both hands. Grasp both arms above your head with your hands facing away from each other. The tube should be behind your head.

2. Pull down with your arms until your arms are at shoulder height.
3. Return to starting position. Complete 3 to 15 repetitions. Complete 1 to 3 sets.

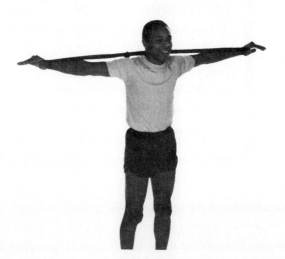

15

EVALUATING EXERCISE PROGRAMS

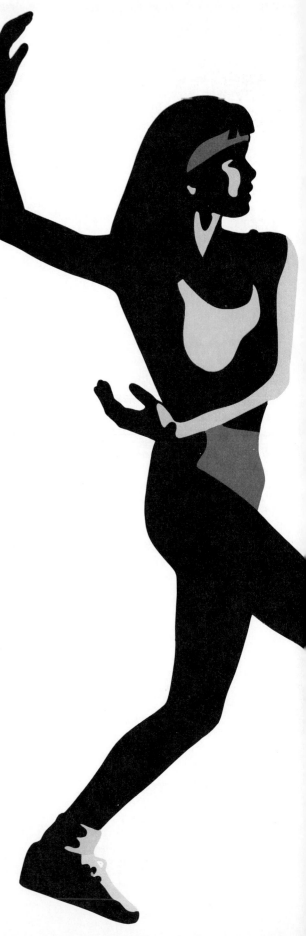

You already know that regular physical activity contributes to your good health and well-being. You also know that no one activity or exercise is best for everyone. An individual's choice of physical activity is based on such factors as age, interests, present physical ability, and fitness goals. In this chapter you will learn about different kinds of exercise programs, how to plan an exercise program, and how to evaluate exercise programs. Exercise and activities can be divided into three groups—planned exercise programs, general exercise programs, and sports and other activities.

PLANNED EXERCISE PROGRAMS

Exercise programs you read about in magazines and books or see on television and videotapes are examples of planned programs. These programs are made up of workouts that are recommended for people of specific ages or fitness levels. Some planned programs are progressive. They include several workouts, each one more difficult than the previous one. As your fitness improves, you progress to the more advanced workout plan.

Planned programs have both advantages and disadvantages. A planned program usually does not require additional planning on your part. It might include appealing music, attractive pictures, or video-taped examples. However, there are three potential problems: program are often too easy, they are often not planned by fitness experts and might contain potentially harmful exercises, or these programs might concentrate on only one or two areas of fitness. Continue reading to find out about effective planned exercise programs.

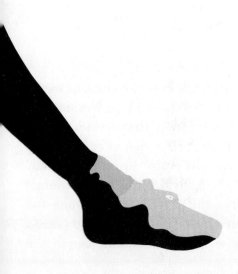

CALISTHENICS *Calisthenics* are exercises done using your own body parts or body weight as resistance. Push-ups, sit-ups, and side-leg raises are examples of calisthenics. A calisthenics workout usually includes strength, muscular endurance, and flexibility exercises. Calisthenics can supplement sports or general exercise programs that build cardiovascular fitness. They are sometimes called "home exercises" because they can be done at home without special equipment. A home calisthenics program is described on pages 194 and 195.

AEROBIC DANCE *Aerobic dance* is a combination of dance steps and calisthenics done to music. In recent years, it has become popular to refer to aerobic dance and similar types of dance exercise as "aerobics." While dance exercise is one form of aerobics, other activities such as jogging, swimming, and walking can also qualify.

Aerobic-dance instruction is available at community recreation departments, health clubs and on videotapes. Recently, *low-impact aerobics* was developed to lessen the risk of joint and muscle injury through repeated hopping and jumping. Low-impact aerobics keeps one foot in contact with the floor at all times. A sample aerobic-dance routine is described on pages 74 and 75.

INTERVAL TRAINING When used for cardiovascular fitness, *interval training* might consist of fast running of short distances followed by a short walk or jog, rather than running or jogging long distances at a slow pace. Interval training is anaerobic rather than aerobic. While interval training can be performed in different ways, the best program is one based on your personal fitness needs. A sample program is shown here:
1. Jog slowly for 2 minutes.
2. Run 220 yards at 80 percent of your fastest speed or faster.
3. Walk 110 yards. Then jog 110 yards.
4. Repeat the above sequence three times.
5. Run 440 yards at 60 to 80 percent of your fastest speed.
6. Walk 220 yards. Then jog 220 yards.
7. Repeat the above sequence twice.

PARCOURSE A *parcourse* usually has 10 to 20 exercise stations located at least 100 yards, and up to 400 yards, apart. The exercise stations are permanently installed and are outdoors rather than indoors. Simple exercise equipment is located at each station. A sign at each station suggests the number of repetitions of each exercise to be completed. "PAR" is an acronym for the number of "physical activity repetitions" to be completed. There are usually several "PARs" listed—one for beginners, another for regular exercisers, and a third for advanced exercisers. After completing the exercise, the participant jogs to the next station.

A parcourse can be established in a park, on schoolgrounds, or anywhere that provides a large space. If your community has a parcourse, try it out. If not, you might want to help establish one.

ORIENTEERING *Orienteering* combines walking, jogging, and map-reading skills. It is usually done in a rural area and might include hiking through somewhat rugged terrain. Each participant leaves from a starting point every few minutes so that he or she cannot follow the person ahead. Each participant has a compass and a map that describes a course from one to ten miles. The compass is used to help locate several "checkpoints" that are marked by flags or other identification. At each checkpoint, the participant marks a card to indicate that the checkpoint has been located. The object is to cover the course in as little time as possible.

OTHER PROGRAMS Aqua dynamics, Cooper's aerobics, continuous rhythmical exercise, circuit training, and weight training are among other planned exercise programs. Information on each of these programs can be found on these pages: aqua dynamics, pages 134-135; Cooper's aerobics, pages 58-59; continuous rhythmical exercise, pages 160-161; circuit training, pages 40-41; weight training, pages 90-91.

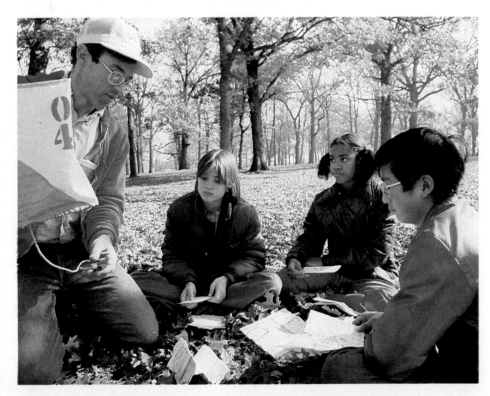

Orienteering is one of many planned exercise programs.

GENERAL EXERCISE PROGRAMS

You already know that planned programs usually contain workouts that include many different exercises done one after another. Sports are games with specific rules. However, general exercise programs are neither planned programs nor sports. General exercises, such as swimming, walking, jogging, and bicycling, are among the most popular in the United States partly because they do not require a lot of skill or special equipment.

Read about and try the exercises described here. Once you have tried them, you can plan your own general exercise workouts. Daily workouts can vary; different combinations of general exercise workouts can be used in a total exercise program. Use the FIT Formula as you plan. Remember to warm-up before, and cool-down after, a workout.

BICYCLING Recreational bicycling is among the most popular activities for developing and maintaining fitness. Depending on the route and pace selected, bicycling can contribute to cardiovascular fitness and development of muscular endurance. A sample bicycling program is described below.

1. Ride on a predetermined 3-mile course. Beginners should select a course that is as level as possible. Experienced bicyclists should plan a route that includes equal amounts of uphill and downhill riding.

2. Start with a slower pace, gradually working your way to your target zone. Maintain a steady pace throughout the majority of the ride. Slowly reduce your pace near the end of your course to help you cool down. Try to complete the course in 18 minutes or less, if possible.

DANCE Dancing is the world's first form of body language—a form that strives to let the body speak for itself. Being one of the oldest art forms, dancing has always been an expression by people of various cultures. Some forms of dance can be enjoyable as well as excellent forms of exercise. Modern dance can help build health-related fitness. Ballet develops strength and flexibility. Square dancing can contribute to skill-related fitness as well as cardiovascular endurance.

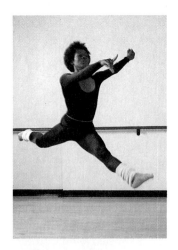

Ballet is only one form of dance.

HIKING AND BACKPACKING Hiking is particularly enjoyable because it is an outdoor activity that can be done independently or with others. Depending on the terrain and route chosen, hiking can contribute to muscle development and cardiovascular fitness. Most county, state, and national parks have a wide variety of scenic trails for hikers of all levels of experience. Inexperienced hikers should stay with well-marked, established trails. More experienced hikers might hike in less-familiar areas, but should carry a map, compass, and water supply with them.

While hiking is usually a one-day experience, backpacking is often a several-day venture. You carry your food, shelter, and other supplies in a pack on your back. Though both hiking and backpacking can build fitness, they also require an established level of fitness. Before you begin, do some walking, jogging, and/or other exercises to build up muscular endurance in your legs. Hike short distances regularly for a few weeks before planning a backpacking trip. Wear hiking boots and loose-fitting clothing for comfort and to protect yourself from possible injury. "Break in" your hiking boots before you use them for backpacking.

SPEEDPLAY A popular form of exercise in Europe is *speedplay*. This activity includes walking, fast walking, slow jogging, fast jogging, calisthenics, and occasional sprints. Rather than continually jogging at the same pace, speedplay allows you to enjoy the scenery and vary your pace. A sample program is described below. If possible, choose a scenic area with a slightly hilly terrain.
1. Walk for one minute.
2. Jog for two minutes.
3. Run 200 yards at approximately 75 percent of your fastest speed.
4. Complete these calisthenics without resting between exercises:
   —3 to 5 bent knee sit-ups
   —3 to 5 side leg raises with each leg
   —3 to 5 push-ups or knee push-ups
5. Repeat steps 1, 2, and 3.
6. Walk for two minutes.

If this routine is too difficult, walk instead of jog, when necessary. If the routine is too easy, repeat each activity.

HAVE YOU HEARD?
One of the first documented studies on running and mental health was done by John Greist at the University of Wisconsin in 1976. The study showed that jogging offered a better treatment for depression than psychotherapy.

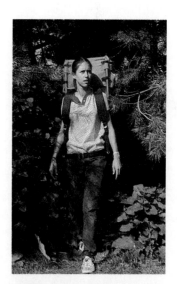

Build muscular endurance in your legs before backpacking.

SWIMMING Swimming is a good form of exercise even if you do not swim competitively. You can use a variety of strokes, such as the backstroke, breaststroke, sidestroke, and a kickboard, with the sample program described here. Some strokes and kicks are described on pages 212-213.

1. Slowly swim 2 lengths of a 25-yard or 25-meter pool or 1 length of a 50-yard or 50-meter pool in 30 to 40 seconds.

2. Get out of the pool, and walk back to the other end of the pool.

3. Repeat this swimming/walking procedure 8 times.

WALKING Brisk walking can improve muscle endurance and cardiovascular fitness in people of all ages. Walking is especially good for older people and people who, for medical or other reasons, should not run or jog. If you regularly walk for exercise, you might buy a pair of shoes designed for this activity. A sample walking program is described below:

1. Plan a 1½-mile walking course that includes walking uphill and downhill, preferably in a scenic area. You might work with your classmates to plan several different routes.

2. Try to walk the course in 20 minutes or less. Start slowly, increasing your pace as you walk. As you near the end of the course, slow your pace to help you cool down.

OTHER PROGRAMS Jogging and jumping rope are among other general exercise programs. Information on these programs can be found on these pages: jogging, pages 30-31; jumping rope, pages 146-147.

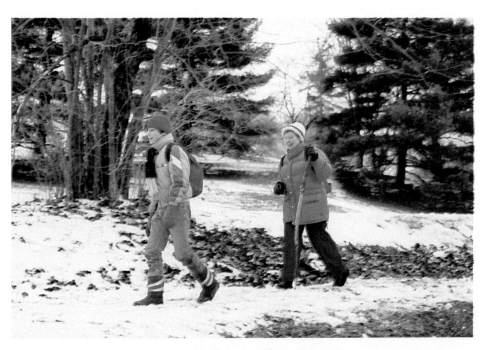

Brisk walking improves cardiovascular fitness.

BENEFITS OF EXERCISE PROGRAMS

Before choosing exercise programs that are best for you, study this chart. It lists the benefits gained from each exercise program. You will learn about the benefits of sports and other activities in Chapter 16.

Health-Related Benefits of Exercise Programs

	Develops Cardiovascular Fitness	Develops Strength	Develops Muscular Endurance	Develops Flexibility	Helps Control Body Fatness
Planned Programs					
Aerobic Dance ★ ▪	excellent	fair	good	good	excellent
Aqua Dynamics ★	good	fair	good	fair	good
Continuous Rhythmical Exercise ★	excellent	fair	excellent	good	excellent
Cooper's Aerobics ★	excellent	fair	good	poor	excellent
Circuit Training ★	fair	good	excellent	good	fair
Fitness Calisthenics ★	poor	fair/good	good/excellent	excellent	poor
Interval Training ★ ▪	excellent	fair	good	poor	excellent
Orienteering ★	excellent	poor	good	poor	excellent
Parcourse ★ ▪	good	good	excellent	good	good
Weight Training ★	poor	excellent	good	poor	fair
General Exercise Programs					
Bicycling ★	excellent	fair	good	poor	excellent
Dance					
ballet ▪	fair/good	good	good	excellent	fair/good
modern ▪	fair/good	fair	good	excellent	fair/good
social ★	fair/good	poor	fair	fair	fair/good
Hiking/Backpacking ★ ▪	good	fair/good	excellent	fair	good
Jogging ★	excellent	poor	good	poor	excellent
Rope Jumping ★	good	poor	good	poor	good
Speedplay ★ ▪	excellent	fair	good	poor	excellent
Swimming ★	excellent	fair	good	fair	excellent
Walking ★	good	poor	fair	poor	good

★ Denotes lifetime sport.

▪ Denotes fitness needed to prevent injury.

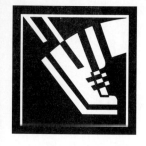

ACTIVITY

EVALUATING PROGRAMS AND ACTIVITIES

WORKSHEET 15-1

Use worksheet 15-1 to evaluate your chosen exercise programs and activities.

One way to evaluate an exercise program or activity is to determine which fitness areas the program or activity emphasizes. Does it work on cardiovascular fitness? strength? muscular endurance? flexibility? controlling body fat? Next, think about the program or activity in terms of your own needs. Does it meet your needs? If not, how might you supplement the program or activity? Then try the program or activity for a few weeks. Finally, ask yourself if you really enjoyed what you were doing. You might eventually discontinue an exercise program if you consider it a chore rather than something enjoyable.

Use worksheet 15-1 to evaluate one or more exercise programs or activities that were described in this chapter. You might compare your results with your classmates to see if you have programs or activities on which you can work together.

PLANNING YOUR OWN WORKOUT

You have read about and tried exercise programs with workouts developed by other people. You can plan your own workout by following these guidelines:

● **Consider all parts of fitness.** Plan exercises for all five parts of health-related fitness, if possible.

● **Avoid dangerous exercise.** Avoid dangerous exercises, such as those described in Chapter 2, when planning your workout.

● **Alternate muscle groups.** Alternating muscle groups means using different muscles from one exercise to another. Avoid performing consecutive exercises that work the same muscle group. For example, if you use your arms in one exercise, your next exercise should work a different muscle group, such as your legs.

● **Consider your own fitness level.** Your workout exercises should be challenging, but not too difficult. Do not include exercises that you cannot do properly. Consider the results of your self-evaluations so that you include exercises that you really need.

● **Vary your workouts.** Include different exercises in your workout to keep it interesting. From time to time, change the exercises.

CHAPTER REVIEW

MULTIPLE CHOICE

Choose the letter of the best answer.

1. A planned exercise program that consists of exercise stations located 100 yards to 400 yards apart is (a) orienteering. (b) speedplay. (c) parcourse. (d) calisthenics.
2. The cardiovascular benefits of swimming are (a) excellent. (b) fair. (c) good. (d) poor.
3. Which is an example of a planned exercise program? (a) orienteering (b) hiking (c) bicycling (d) walking
4. Exercises done using your own body parts or body weight as resistance are (a) low-impact aerobics. (b) calisthenics. (c) high-impact aerobics. (d) cardiovascular exercises.
5. Which program combines walking, jogging, and map-reading skills? (a) interval training (b) speedplay (c) orienteering (d) parcourse
6. General exercise programs (a) require much skill or special equipment. (b) are planned by fitness experts. (c) consist of games with specific rules. (d) are neither planned programs nor sports.
7. Which is an example of a general exercise program? (a) aerobic dance (b) interval training (c) swimming (d) weight training
8. An exercise that is especially good for older people is (a) jogging. (b) running. (c) jumping rope. (d) brisk walking.
9. Interval training (a) is aerobic rather than anaerobic. (b) is anaerobic rather than aerobic. (c) is neither aerobic nor anaerobic. (d) combines dance steps and calisthenics.
10. Which activity best develops flexibility? (a) swimming (b) modern dancing (c) jogging (d) bicycling

MATCHING

Match the definition in Column I with the term it defines in Column II.

Column I

11. exercises done when you use your own body parts or body weight as resistance
12. activity that includes walking, jogging, calisthenics, and sprints
13. planned exercise program done to music that combines dance steps and calisthenics
14. activity that combines walking, jogging, and map-reading skills
15. planned exercise program that requires you to keep one foot in contact with the floor at all times when dancing

Column II

a. aerobic dance
b. calisthenics
c. low-impact aerobics
d. orienteering
e. speedplay

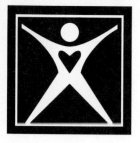

FOCUS ON FITNESS

CALISTHENICS AT HOME

This calisthenics program is planned especially for people your age. It includes a warm-up, a workout, and a cool-down. Use Level 1 if you do not exercise regularly or had a low score on most parts of fitness evaluated earlier. Use Level 2 if you exercise regularly or scored well on earlier evaluations. Use Level 3 after you have exercised for several weeks and notice a significant change in your fitness levels. Substitute exercises from Chapters 6 through 10 to vary the program.

CALISTHENICS AT HOME

Exercise	Repetitions or Length of Time		
	Level 1	Level 2	Level 3
Warm-up			
Calf Stretcher (each leg)	3	3	3
Sitting Windmill	5	10	15
Jog in Place	1–2 min.	2 minutes	2 minutes
Workout			
Knee Dip (each leg)	1–5	6–10	11–15
6-Count Push-up	1–5	6–10	11–15
Cardiovascular Exercise*	1 minute	2 minutes	3 minutes
Knee-to-Nose (each leg)	1–5	6–10	11–15
Trunk Curl	1–5	6–15	16–25
Cardiovascular Exercise*	1 minute	2 minutes	3 minutes
Towel Squeeze	1–5	6–10	6–10
Toe Raise	1–5	6–10	11–15
Cardiovascular Exercise*	1 minute	2 minutes	3 minutes
Cool-down			
Shake-down	1 minute	1 minute	1 minute
Sitting Windmill	5	10	15
Calf Stretcher	3	3	3

*Choose one of the cardiovascular exercises you have learned.

CALF STRETCHER

● See page 10 for directions for this exercise.

SITTING WINDMILL

1. Sit with your feet apart, your hands held sideward at shoulder level, and palms down. Bend knees slightly.
2. Bend and twist your trunk. Touch your right hand to your left toe.
3. Return to starting positon and repeat, touching your left hand to your right toe.
Caution: Do exercise slowly.

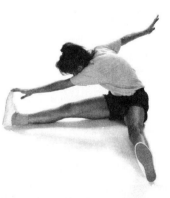

JOG IN PLACE

● See page 21 for directions for this exercise.

KNEE DIP

1. Stand on your right foot while holding on to a chair. Squat down. Continue bending down until your right knee is bent at a 90° angle.
2. Return to starting position. Repeat with your other leg.

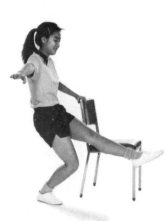

6-COUNT PUSH UP

1. Stand straight with your arms at your side.
2. Squat, bending knees no more than 90°. Place palms flat on the floor at about shoulder-width apart and your arms between your knees.
3. Thrust your legs backward into push-up positon. *Caution:* Do not arch your back. Keep back and legs straight.
4. Continue to keep your back and legs straight. Bend your arms at your elbows until your chest touches the floor.
5. Straighten your arms. Return to push-up position.
6. Return to half-squat position, and then to starting position. *Note:* If you cannot do a push-up, ask your teacher to demonstrate a modified push-up.

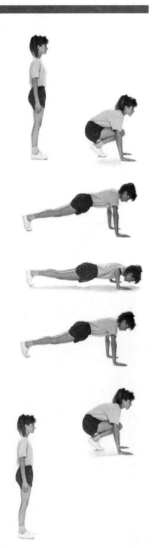

KNEE-TO-NOSE

● See page 21 for directions for this exercise.

TRUNK CURL

● See page 55 for directions for this exercise.

TOWEL SQUEEZE

1. Fold a bath towel into fourths and roll it into a cylinder. The cylinder should be small enough to get your hands around when you squeeze it.
2. Hold the towel in both hands with your palms up. Grasp the towel with your left hand, tightening your grip as much as possible. Hold for 2 seconds.
3. Release and repeat with your other hand.

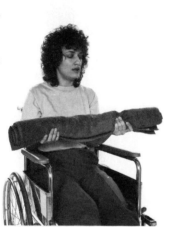

TOE RAISE

1. Stand on a stair, large book, or block of wood. Put your weight on the balls of your feet. Keep your heels raised.
2. Lower your heels to the floor.
3. Repeat raising and lowering your heels.

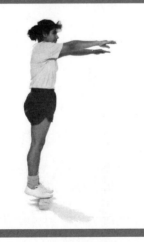

SHAKE DOWN

1. Stand with your body fully relaxed. Walk around with very long steps to stretch your leg and hamstring muscles.
2. At the same time, shake your arms and hands along your sides. Gently roll your head in half circles.

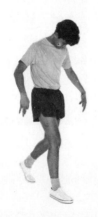

16

FITNESS
AND SPORTS

CHAPTER OBJECTIVES

After reading this chapter, you should be able to:

✔ Discuss factors involved in selecting sports.

✔ Discuss which sports develop different parts of fitness.

✔ Evaluate different sports.

✔ Choose a lifetime sport.

Not too many years ago, most people had to work very hard to survive. They put in long hours at their jobs, which left them with very little leisure time. A twelve-hour work day was not uncommon. As a rule, young people as well as adults had little free time because the labor force included many children and teenagers.

Today, machines do much of the work that people used to do by hand. Thus, leisure time has increased. Now, people of all ages have more free time for recreation, sports, and other enjoyable activities.

Sports are an important leisure-time activity for many teenagers. After school, for example, young people participate in competitive sports such as football, soccer, basketball, wrestling, volleyball, track, and baseball.

Many adults also enjoy sports. However, most are no longer involved in team sports such as the ones mentioned above. Instead, they have learned other sports—ones that are suitable for all age groups. In this chapter, you will investigate such sports and might become interested in learning one or more of these sports. Such sports can provide you with enjoyment now and throughout the adult years of your life.

SPORTS FOR ALL AGES

Recently, adults were surveyed to find out how their interests in sports had changed through the years. Results of the survey indicated that the sports adults played most often when they were in school were baseball, basketball, and football. However, none of these sports was listed among the most popular activities currently played by the same people. Instead, they now preferred bowling, tennis, and golf.

Team sports are good activities for teenagers. If you are involved in a varsity or an intramural team sport, you know how much fun these activities can be. In addition, these sports help you keep fit.

Nevertheless, consider learning other sports in addition to the ones you already play. Now is a good time to learn a lifetime sport. A *lifetime sport* is an activity that is suitable for people of all age groups. Activities, such as bowling, tennis, and golf, are good examples of lifetime sports. These sports not only provide adults with enjoyment, they also help them keep fit. If you learn how to play a lifetime sport as a teenager, you are much more likely to continue playing it throughout your adult life.

When you are deciding which lifetime sport to take up, select one you think you might enjoy—one that looks interesting to you. Avoid sports that seem more like work than fun. Many people give up sports, as well as exercise programs, because they have picked an activity that they do not really enjoy.

BENEFITS OF SPORTS

If you were to ask ten different people why they enjoy sports, you might get ten different answers. Some might respond that participating in a sport is a good way to "get away from it all" and have fun. Others might say participating in sports enables them to socialize with friends and meet new people. Finally, many people enjoy sports because it helps them keep fit.

If you plan to use sports as part of your fitness program, choose ones that will help you develop the parts of fitness you want to improve. For good health both today and in the future, build an exercise or conditioning program around your sports activities, and stay with the program on a regular basis.

The table on page 199 lists some health and fitness benefits of various sports. The activities that might be considered lifetime sports are highlighted. Each activity is rated according to how much it can contribute to health and fitness. The ratings are based on vigorous participation in the activity.

If you play less vigorously, expect fewer fitness benefits. For example, badminton played by the official rules provides the benefits listed in the table. On the other hand, playing badminton in your backyard might not provide as many benefits.

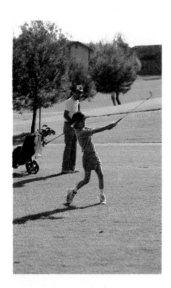

Golf is a lifetime sport.

Health-Related Benefits of Sports

Sport	Develops Cardiovascular Fitness	Develops Strength	Develops Muscular Endurance	Develops Flexibility	Helps Control Body Fatness
Archery ★	poor	fair	poor	poor	poor
Badminton ★	fair	poor	fair	fair	fair
Baseball ▪	poor	poor	poor	poor	poor
Basketball					
half court ★ ▪	fair	poor	fair	poor	fair
vigorous ★ ▪	excellent	poor	good	poor	excellent
Bowling ★	poor	poor	poor	poor	poor
Canoeing ★	fair	poor	fair	poor	fair
Fencing ▪	fair	fair	good	fair	fair
Football ▪	fair	good	fair	poor	fair
Golf (walking) ★	fair	poor	poor	fair	fair
Gymnastics ▪	fair	excellent	excellent	excellent	fair
Handball ★ ▪	good/excellent	poor	good	poor	good/excellent
Horseback Riding ★	poor	poor	poor	poor	poor
Judo/Karate ★ ▪	poor	fair	fair	fair	poor
Mountain Climbing ★ ▪	good	good	good	poor	good
Pool/Billiards ★	poor	poor	poor	poor	poor
Racquetball ★ ▪	good/excellent	poor	good	poor	good/excellent
Rowing, Crew	excellent	fair	excellent	poor	excellent
Sailing ★	poor	poor	poor	poor	poor
Skating					
ice ★ ▪	fair/good	poor	good	poor	fair/good
roller ★ ▪	fair/good	poor	fair	poor	fair/good
Skiing					
cross-country ★ ▪	excellent	fair	good	poor	excellent
downhill ★ ▪	poor	fair	fair	poor	poor
Soccer ▪	excellent	fair	good	fair	excellent
Softball ★ ▪	poor	poor	poor	poor	poor
Surfing ★ ▪	fair	poor	good	fair	fair
Table Tennis ★	poor	poor	poor	poor	poor
Tennis ★ ▪	fair/good	poor	fair	poor	fair/good
Volleyball ★ ▪	fair	fair	poor	poor	fair
Waterskiing ★ ▪	fair	fair	fair	poor	fair

★ Denotes lifetime sport.

▪ Denotes fitness needed to prevent injury.

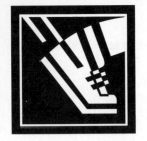

ACTIVITY

CHOOSING YOUR LIFETIME SPORT

WORKSHEET 16-1

Record your results of this activity on worksheet 16-1.

Complete this activity to help you get started with a new sport.

1. Study the table on page 199. Write down a lifetime sport you might like to learn.

2. Use an encyclopedia or other reference books to learn more about this sport. Include ideas such as: when and where it was first played; countries in which this sport is most popular, and so on.

3. Briefly describe the play of the sport: rules, players, and so on.

4. Perform the sport you have chosen in class or at home. Evaluate the sport to see if it is a good choice for you.

FITNESS FOR SPORTS

Just as sports can contribute to good fitness, you also must stay fit to participate actively in sports. A *weekend athlete* is someone who neither exercises nor plays a sport on a regular basis. For example, some people snow ski only once or twice a year, but otherwise do not exercise regularly. Nevertheless, they believe they are fit enough to ski. In fact, these people should exercise regularly for several weeks before skiing to get ready for it and to avoid injury.

Some individuals mistakenly assume that fitness is not necessary for certain sports, especially if the sports do little to build fitness. For instance, softball is not particularly good for developing fitness, but it does requires fitness in order to perform well. A player must sprint between bases, slide into bases, jump to catch a ball, and bat. Each action is likely to result in an injury if the player is not physically fit.

Note the activities on page 199 in which you must be especially fit as to play safely and skillfully. Be fit *before* actively playing a sport that involves the factors listed here. Each item is a condition or action that could cause injury.

1. **Physical contact:** football, wrestling, ice hockey
2. **Fast sprinting:** baseball, softball, soccer
3. **Sudden fast starts and stops:** racquetball, handball, basketball
4. **Vigorous jumping:** basketball, some track-and-field activities
5. **Danger of falling:** skiing, skating
6. **Danger of overstretching muscles:** tennis, football

HAVE YOU HEARD?

Biomechanical principles, or rules that help the human machine function efficiently, can help you play sports. For example, following the principles of running (pg. 30) can help you perform well in basketball, track and field, and soccer.

CHAPTER REVIEW

MULTIPLE CHOICE

Choose the letter of the best answer.

1. Why are sports and activities more important today than they were 100 years ago? (a) more leisure time today (b) more sports to play (c) more sporting equipment available (d) people work longer hours

2. Which sport probably is favored by the largest number of adults? (a) touch football (b) marathon races (c) golf (d) soccer

3. Which is *not* especially a benefit of sports? (a) fitness (b) enjoyment (c) social experience (d) gives resistance to disease

4. Which sport probably is least helpful for building fitness? (a) golf (b) tennis (c) volleyball (d) bowling

5. Which is the basis of the sports ratings in the table on page 199? (a) light activity (b) moderate activity (c) vigorous activity (d) irregular activity

6. You want to control body fatness. Which is probably the best sport for you? (a) soccer (b) archery (c) softball (d) volleyball

7. You want to develop strength. Which sport should you select? (a) golf (b) gymnastics (c) badminton (d) judo

8. Which is the best sport for developing cardiovascular fitness? (a) baseball (b) football (c) cross-country skiing (d) gymnastics

9. Which is the best sport for developing muscular endurance? (a) baseball (b) gymnastics (c) racquetball (d) soccer

10. Which most likely is *least* helpful for developing flexibility? (a) waterskiing (b) soccer (c) golf (d) judo

MATCHING

Match the definition in Column I with the term it defines in Column II.

Column I

11. potential for injury, especially for wrestlers
12. potential for injury, especially for skiiers
13. potential for injury, especially for racquetball players
14. person who does not regularly participate in exercises or sports
15. suitable for people of all ages

Column II

a. falling
b. lifelong sports
c. physical contact
d. sudden fast starts and stops
e. weekend athlete

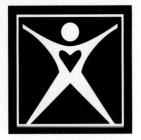

FOCUS ON FITNESS

THE SPORTS STARS EXERCISE PROGRAM

The Sports Stars Exercise Program is designed to help you use sports in your exercise program. The program is based on earning a certain number of stars, or points, per week. You should earn 100 stars per week to build good health-related fitness, especially cardiovascular fitness, if this is your only activity. If you use sports as only a part of your exercise program, you might earn fewer than 100 stars. Follow these guidelines in earning stars:

● **Earn stars at least 3 days per week.** Ideally, you should earn Sports stars 4 to 6 days per week.

● **Build all parts of health-related fitness.** Many sports do not build all parts of fitness. Therefore, you have to exercise to build those parts of fitness not covered by sports. However, if you participate in school varsity sports, you probably do conditioning as well as play the sport. Thus, you probably are building all parts of fitness.

● **Start the Sports Stars Program gradually.** Earn 50 points a week during the first two weeks. Then earn 75 points a week during the third and fourth weeks. Finally, work to earn 100 points a week.

● **The benefits you get from the Sports Stars Program depend on the amount of time and effort you invest in the program.** Stars are based on continuous participation. Do not count the time you rest during an activity.

● **Vary your program.** You can earn 100 stars in any of the sports listed. However, many of the sports are *not* intense enough to build good fitness. Therefore, your program should not be based solely on sports for which you earn 6 or fewer stars per hour. You might earn some stars with these sports, but earn at least 60 stars from more vigorous sports.

● **Remember to warm up and stretch and cool down and stretch.** Warming up before exercise, and cooling down after exercise, helps reduce your risk of injuries.

This chart shows the number of stars you can earn with various exercises. Use the chart to help plan your exercise program.

NUMBER OF STARS EARNED IN SPORTS

Sport	15 minutes	30 minutes	1 hour	2 hours	Comments
Archery	¾	1 ½	3	6	
Badminton					
doubles	1	2	4	8	
singles	3	6	12	24	
Baseball					
recreational	1	2	4	8	
school team	3	6	12	24	team practice
Basketball					
recreational	3	6	12	24	full court
school team	4 ½	9	18	36	team practice
Bowling	¾	1 ½	3	6	
Canoeing	3	6	12	24	continuous paddling
Football					
recreational	2	4	8	16	
school team	4 ½	9	18	36	team practice
Golf	1 ½	3	6	12	walking; steady play
Gymnastics					
school team	3	6	12	24	team practice
Handball	4 ½	9	18	36	steady play
Horseback Riding	1	2	4	8	
Judo or Karate	2	4	8	16	no long breaks
Racquetball	4 ½	9	18	36	steady play
Rowing					
crew team	6	12	24	48	actual rowing time
Skating					
(ice or roller)	3 ½	7	14	28	actual skating time
Skiing					
cross-country	1	16	32	64	actual skiing time
downhill	4 ½	9	18	32	actual skiing time
Soccer					
recreational	4	8	16	32	actual playing time
school team	5	10	20	40	team practice
Softball					
recreational	1	2	4	8	
school team	3	6	12	24	team practice
Tennis					
doubles	2	4	8	16	
singles	3 ½	7	14	28	
Volleyball					
recreational	1	2	4	8	
school team	3	6	12	24	team practice
Wrestling					
school team	5	10	20	40	team practice

17

PLANNING YOUR EXERCISE PROGRAM

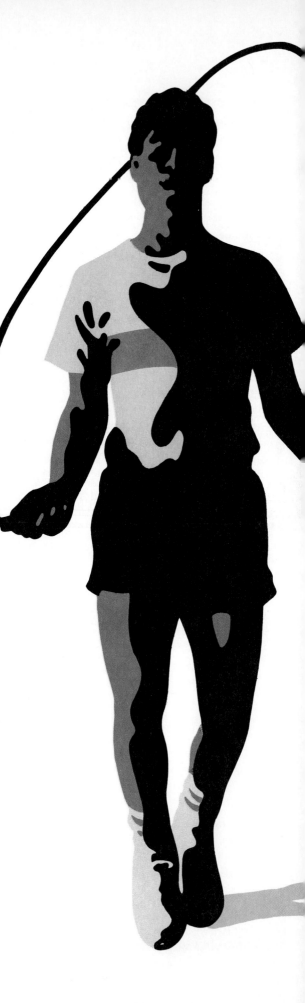

CHAPTER OBJECTIVES

After reading this chapter, you should be able to:

✔ Describe the steps involved in planning a personal exercise program.

✔ List activities to include in a personal exercise program.

✔ Plan a personal exercise program.

You already know that regular activity can help you feel and look good. You know *who* can exercise, *why* exercise is important and *how* to exercise properly. Now you need to decide *what* you are going to do, *when* you are going to do it, and *where* you are going to do it. In this chapter, you will learn how to develop a *personal exercise program*, a weekly exercise plan that you can follow easily to achieve your lifetime fitness goals.

DECIDING WHAT TO DO

You can plan an effective personalized exercise program by following the six steps discussed here. By doing so, you will set reasonable goals, plan how to achieve the goals, and enjoy working to achieve the goals.

Achieving short-term exercise goals will help you meet your long-term physical goals. For example, if your cardiovascular fitness level is marginal, your long-term fitness goal might be to improve your cardiovascular fitness to the good level. Your short-term exercise goal might be to perform an exercise program with cardiovascular exercises for a specific number of weeks. Then you can evaluate your progress with the one-mile run or step test. Remember that it takes time to improve your fitness through exercise.

WORKSHEET 17-1

Use worksheet 17-1 to record your selections for your personalized exercise program.

STEP 1 Use worksheet 17-1 or copy the chart shown here. List the health-related ratings you scored on the self-evaluations you completed in Chapters 6, 7, 8, 9, and 10 to help you. Refer to the page numbers given on the chart to find these self-evaluations. Indicate your rating by placing an "X" in the appropriate box under each fitness part.

Step 1: Health-Related Benefits

Fitness Rating	Cardiovascular Fitness (pages 69 and 70)	Strength (page 79)	Muscular Endurance (pages 96 and 97)	Flexibility (pages 108 and 109)	Body Fatness (pages 127 and 128)
High Performance					
Good					
Marginal					
Low					

STEP 2 Continue using worksheet 17-1 or copy the chart below. List the activities *you* enjoy. Use the information from Chapters 15 and 16 to help you select activities from planned exercise programs, general exercise programs, or sports. When selecting activities, remember to consider those that match your skill-related fitness.

Use the chart in Chapter 15 to find the ratings of health-related benefits for your activities. Mark the appropriate boxes on your chart, using these letters: E-excellent; G-good; F-fair; P-poor.

Step 2: Health-Related Benefits

Activities I Enjoy	Cardiovascular Fitness	Strength	Muscular Endurance	Flexibility	Body Fatness

STEP 3 Now compare the benefits of the activities you enjoy with your ratings in the self-evaluations. Some of your activities probably improve parts of fitness that you should improve; others might further develop parts of fitness in which you already do well. Decide which fitness parts you want to improve. You are the one who determines how high a rating you want for each fitness part.

Select those activities you think you would like to include in your exercise program. Write them on your chart under "Activities to Improve Fitness." Also include those exercises you have previously listed as enjoyable.

You might find that the activities you enjoy do not build all parts of health-related fitness. You might need to include extra activities to meet your fitness needs. Plan a workout that includes those parts of fitness not covered by your activities. For example, you might include fitness calisthenics, an aerobic dance, or weight-training in your workout if your activities do not build all health-related fitness parts. List each activity's fitness benefits next to its name. You can write several fitness benefits beside one activity since some activities benefit several parts of fitness.

Step 3: Activities to Improve Fitness

Planned Programs	Fitness Benefits
☐ Aerobic Dance	
☐ Aqua Dynamics	
☐ Circuit Training	
☐ Continuous Rhythmical Exercises	
☐ Cooper's Aerobics	
☐ Fitness Calisthenics	
☐ Interval Training	
☐ Orienteering	
☐ Parcourse	

General Exercise Programs	Fitness Benefits
☐ Backpacking	
☐ Bicycling	
☐ Dancing	
☐ Hiking	
☐ Jogging	
☐ Rope Jumping	
☐ Swimming	
☐ Walking	

Sports	Fitness Benefits
☐ Archery	
☐ Badminton	
☐ Baseball	
☐ Bowling	
☐ Canoeing	
☐ Fencing	
☐ Football	
☐ Golf	
☐ Gymnastics	
☐ Handball	
☐ Horseback Riding	

☐ Judo
☐ Karate
☐ Mountain Climbing

☐ Racquetball/Paddleball

☐ Rowing
☐ Sailing
☐ Skating
☐ Skiing
☐ Soccer
☐ Softball
☐ Table Tennis

☐ Tennis
☐ Volleyball
☐ Waterskiing

☐ Wrestling

STEP 4 Make a list of the activities you will include in your program. Include activities that you enjoy from Step 2, and those that you need for building all parts of health-related fitness from Step 3. List the activities on a sheet of paper or use the appropriate place on the worksheet.

STRUCTURING YOUR EXERCISE PROGRAM

Follow step 5 and step 6 to structure your exercise program.

STEP 5 With your list of activities you will include in your exercise program, you can decide when and where you will exercise. Use the information below to help you plan your exercise program.

● **Choosing Days** You already know that you should exercise at least 3 days per week to achieve and maintain fitness. Decide which days you will exercise. Pick at least 3 days of the week during which it would be easiest and most convenient for you to exercise. You might choose Monday, Wednesday, and Friday. You might choose Sunday, Tuesday, and Thursday. You might decide to exercise every other day so that you exercise 3 days one week and 4 days the next week.

Remember that exercise for some parts of fitness, such as strength, should not be done every day. Some people rotate the parts of fitness they work on each day. In other words, they might exercise every day, but work on different parts of fitness on different days. Review the FIT formula charts in Chapters 6, 7, 8, 9, and 10 before you decide on which days of the week to exercise.

● **Choosing Times** At what time of day will you exercise? Will it be early morning? before your evening meal? later in the evening? Some health experts recommend exercise the first thing in the morning because you are fresh and ready to go. Other specialists feel that evening exercise can help you unwind from the stresses of the day. In fact, your best time is when you most enjoy exercising—a time when you are not likely to be interrupted. Keep in mind that you might complete different activities at different times of the day.

Take time to plan an exercise program.

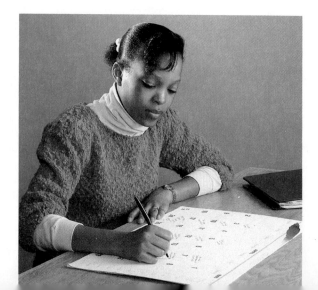

STEP 6 Now you are ready to write your program. On a sheet of paper, list your warm-up exercises. Chapter 2 includes information about planning a warm-up. Chapter 9 includes stretching exercises that might be included in a warm-up. Include exercises that stretch the muscles that you will use while exercising. You might plan more than one warm-up to vary your program.

Now list the activities you will do in each workout session. If you plan special exercises, include them throughout your workout. If you play sports, include practice as part of your program. Remember to include cardiovascular exercises, and to continue them long enough to raise your heart rate to your desired level.

Finally, list your cool-down exercises. Remember to include stretching exercises for muscle cool-down and a cardiovascular cool-down.

The sample weekly program shows you how to write a program. The person making this program wanted to lose body fat and improve cardiovascular fitness. The person did not have high skill-related fitness scores, so jogging was chosen. The person enjoys tennis and, through practice, built enough skill to enjoy playing the game. Special exercises were included to maintain strength, muscular endurance, and flexibility.

● **Choosing Where to Exercise** Your own home is usually the most convenient place in which to exercise. Researchers have found that if people cannot exercise at home, they are most likely to exercise regularly if the location is convenient.

Weekly Exercise Plan for <u>Oct.</u> <u>20</u> **to** <u>Oct.</u> <u>27</u>

            Month   Day   Month   Day

Day	Activity	Time of Day	How Long?	Specific Exercises
M O N	jogging calisthenics	7:30 a.m. 10:00 p.m.	20 min. 10 min	I will do: active side stretches, passive toe reach, 3 sets of bent-knee sit ups and 3 sets of simple push-ups
T U E	tennis calisthenics	4:00 p.m. 4:45 p.m.	45 min. 10 min.	I will do: active side stretches passive toe reach side leg raises
W E D	jogging calisthenics	7:30 a.m. 10:00 p.m.	20 min. 10 min.	Same calisthenics as Monday

---

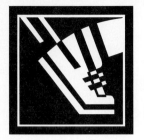

ACTIVITY

EVALUATING YOUR EXERCISE PLAN

WORKSHEET 17-2

Use worksheet 17-2 to evaluate your exercise plan and physical fitness goals.

Try your one-week plan either in class or on your own. Then answer the questions on your worksheet to evaluate your plan. Use these guidelines to help you continue your exercise plan:

● Modify your exercise program until you have a program that you like and can stay with. Your instructor might have extra sheets for planning a one-week exercise plan. If not, make up your own form.

● You will probably want to vary your plan from time to time to keep it interesting and enjoyable.

● Evaluate yourself occasionally to see if your weekly plan is still helping you to meet your fitness goals.

Various factors can cause your exercise program to change from time to time. These factors include the seasonal changes in weather, changes in your schedule, sport seasons, and changes in your fitness needs and interests. Review your plan and revise it when necessary.

Remember that exercise should be fun. Feel free to change your mind from time to time. Sometimes you will be more active than you had planned. At other times you might be less active than you intended to be. Just keep your goal in mind—exercise on a regular basis to stay fit and enjoy life.

Remember that exercise should be enjoyable.

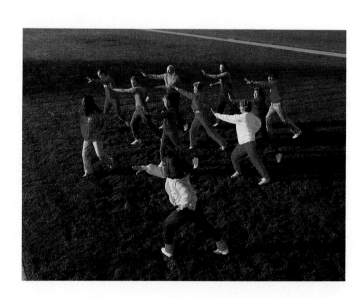

CHAPTER REVIEW

MULTIPLE CHOICE

Choose the letter of the best answer.

1. In planning a personal exercise program, you should (a) exercise only when you feel like it. (b) set reasonable goals. (c) include only activities that you enjoy. (d) ignore activities that you dislike.

2. A person should develop a personal exercise plan (a) on a weekly basis. (b) to last for a month. (c) one day at a time. (d) to last a lifetime.

3. The first step in planning an exercise program is to (a) choose enjoyable activities. (b) decide where to exercise. (c) list your health-related ratings. (d) list each activity.

4. When you list activities that you enjoy, you should (a) list only activities that you do well. (b) also consider those that match your skill-related fitness. (c) never change your mind. (d) choose aerobics.

5. In step 3 of your personal exercise plan, (a) choose only activities that you enjoy. (b) select only activities that you do well. (c) include activities that build all parts of health-related fitness. (d) exercise daily.

6. An exercise plan should include (a) all parts of fitness every day. (b) activities for Mondays, Wednesdays, and Fridays. (c) activities for 5 days each week. (d) a schedule that is easy and convenient.

7. The best time to exercise is (a) when you most enjoy exercising (b) in the morning. (c) after dinner. (d) after school.

8. Warm-up exercises (a) need not be listed in a personal exercise program. (b) should never vary. (c) should be listed as part of an exercise plan. (d) build strength.

9. Cool-down exercises (a) help you lose body fat. (b) build strength. (c) can be omitted. (d) should include stretching exercises and a cardiovascular cool-down.

10. As you evaluate your exercise plan (a) do not change it. (b) modify it until you have a program you can stay with. (c) compare it with someone else's plan. (d) ask your teacher to change it.

MATCHING

Match the definition in Column I with the term it defines in Column II.

Column I

11. a weekly exercise plan to help achieve lifetime fitness goals
12. exercises to stretch muscles before a workout
13. what self-evaluations show

Column II

a. warm-up
b. health-related fitness ratings
c. personal exercise program

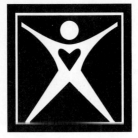

FOCUS ON FITNESS

SWIMMING

People of all ages swim for fun and fitness. Swimming improves cardiovascular fitness and helps develop muscle endurance and coordination. It also is less stressful to your joints than running, jogging, and similar activities since the water keeps you bouyant. Some basic strokes and kicks are discussed here.

When you have learned some of the strokes and kicks, swim for 15 minutes, continuously if possible. If you have not yet learned to swim, exercise for 15 minutes by walking or jogging in the water or use one of the kicks while holding onto the side of the pool or a kickboard.

FRONT CRAWL

1. Move your arms in a steady, circular motion while doing flutter kick. As one hand recovers forward above the water, the other hand pulls beneath the water.

2. Breathe by turning your head to one side just as the hand on that side passes your leg. Inhale through your mouth. Exhale through your mouth or nose while keeping your face in the water.

FLUTTER KICK

1. Alternately move your legs up and down with a slightly relaxed bend at your knees.
2. Power comes from your upper legs. Propulsion comes from your feet as if kicking mud off your feet.

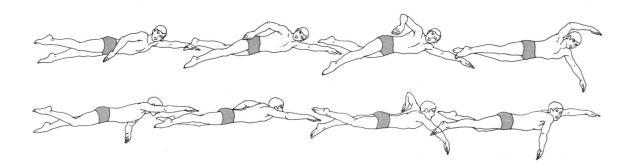

BACKSTROKE

1. Perform the backstroke, or back crawl, as you lie on your back. It is a restful stroke because your face is always out of the water, making breathing easier.

2. As in the front crawl, your arms alternately move in a steady, circular motion in and out of the water while your legs flutter kick.

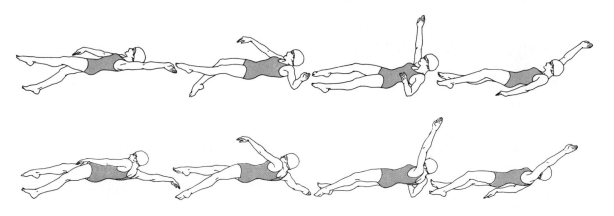

BREASTSTROKE

1. Begin with your face in the water, your arms and legs fully extended, and your palms facing outward. Then sweep out your arms as your hands pull downward and outward.
2. Continue to circle your hands and bring them together under your chin. As your hands begin to push down, lift your head for a breath.
3. Again extend your arms and legs, and glide forward. Make a breaststroke kick at the end of the stroke as your arms extend for a glide.

BREASTSTROKE KICK

1. Begin with your legs fully extended and your toes pointed. Bring your heels toward your hips, just under the surface of the water.
2. As your feet near your hips, bend your knees and extend them outward. Turn your ankles so your toes also point outward.
3. Without pausing, push your feet backward. Squeeze your legs together until your toes again point back.

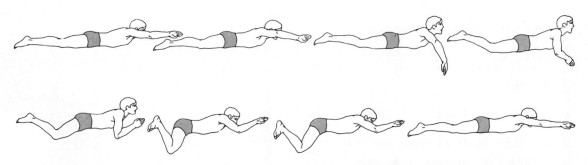

All swimming illustrations pages 212, 213 from the *World Book Encyclopedia.* © 1989 World Book, Inc.

OTHER STROKES You might want to discuss with your instructor how to do these additional strokes and kicks: sidestroke, butterfly stroke, dolphin kick, scissors kick.

18

FITNESS AND YOUR FUTURE

CHAPTER OBJECTIVES

After reading this chapter, you should be able to:

✔ Discuss the term "fitness for life."

✔ List goals to help you stay fit and healthy throughout your life.

✔ Explain what you can do to achieve your fitness goals.

If you think about it, the title of this book has several meanings. One way to interpret "Fitness for Life" is that you need to be fit in order to stay alive. You probably have heard the expression "survival of the fittest." It is often used to explain why some plants and animals survive, while others disappear from the earth. The fittest survive because they are stronger and better adapted to their environment. Because of advances in medical science, human beings sometimes live very many years without being particularly fit. Nevertheless, humans' chances of survival are certainly higher if they are physically fit.

You also might consider the title to mean that life is more than simply survival. You can enjoy life more because you feel better and look better. Both physical health and mental health play an important part in whether or not you have a long and enjoyable life.

Finally, you might think of "fitness for life" as meaning fitness for a lifetime. Being fit for a lifetime is a commitment you must make if you want to get the most from each day of your life. Being fit is not a guarantee that you always will feel good. However, you will feel better if you are fit than if you are not fit. In this chapter, you will learn the importance of maintaining good fitness throughout your life.

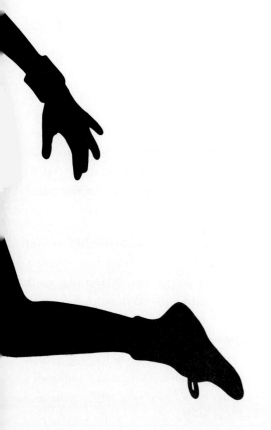

FITNESS FOR TODAY AND TOMORROW

When you were an infant or small child, other people cared for your physical needs. Similarly, medical experts help care for your physical needs if you are ill or injured. However, most of the time you are pretty much in charge of your own body. You select the food you eat to nourish it; you decide how much exercise and rest to give your body; you choose whether or not to abuse your body with drugs or other substances.

Have you ever wondered what you will look or act like when you are an adult? What kind of person do you hope to become? Pretend you have stepped into a "time machine" that allows you to see images of yourself as you would like to be in the future. After one year, you have matured a little and, perhaps, are taller. You have developed further. Your eyes are bright, your posture is erect, and you have learned new physical skills. Next, imagine yourself as a college graduate or as an adult holding a job. Both images show that you are a strong, attractive adult. Then, visualize the way you want to look and feel when you are your parents' ages. Finally, consider an image of yourself as a fit, healthy grandparent with an optimistic attitude toward life. Can these images become a reality? If you hold to your fitness goals, you will be doing all you can to make them come true!

People must accept the aging process, but they need not become less fit as they age. Remember that fitness helps provide good physical and mental health—qualities needed for a happy, productive life.

SETTING YOUR GOALS A Chinese philosopher once said, "A journey of a thousand miles begins with a single step." You can apply this ancient saying to a lifetime fitness goal. For instance, you cannot become as fit and trim as an Olympic athlete overnight. That goal is, in a sense, "a thousand miles away." Today, however, you can take that first step toward your goal. You can continue taking one step at a time, until you reach your goal. Finally, you can *stay* fit in the same way you got there—one step at a time and one day at a time.

KEEPING TO YOUR PLAN A goal of lifelong fitness probably is not your only focus in life. Other goals, such as your education, career, and so on, also compete for your time and attention. Attaining your goals requires self-discipline. Use the guidelines listed here to help you develop and maintain your self-discipline for fitness:

● **Get a support group.** A *fitness support group* includes friends or relatives who provide the encouragement you need to help you attain your fitness goal. Often, the people who exercise with you are members of your support group. A support group can help you when you are tempted to skip your exercises or not eat well.

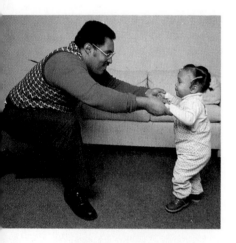

Infants and young children need care and guidance.

People are not supportive if they discourage your efforts to stay healthy by tempting you to indulge yourself. When people give you unreliable advice, tell them that you want to stay with your goal and that you would appreciate their help in doing so.

- **Join a club or group activity.** You are more likely to stay with your exercise program if you have a commitment to other people. Perhaps you might join a cycling club, hiking club, or swim club. You might enjoy an organization such as Junior Achievement or a community recreation program. Also, you might consider joining an organization that offers programs suitable for the whole family, such as a YMCA, YWCA, or church group.
- **Check out summer sports or fitness programs.** Some universities and community colleges sponsor summer sports or fitness programs for young people. Check your local newspapers or call your community's recreation department. You probably can find an activity that will fit your needs and be enjoyable to you.
- **Create a special place to work out.** You do not need to go to a gym or pay to use health club facilities. Consider working with your family and friends to set up an exercise room in your garage, basement, or spare room. The room might include an area for aerobic exercise and homemade weights. If you live in a region where the climate limits outdoor activity, you might buy a bicycle trainer to convert your bicycle to a stationary bicycle for indoor use.
- **Build regular activity into your daily life.** Walk the dog. Wash and wax the family car. Mow the lawn. Walk, jog, or cycle to school. If possible, get off the bus early and walk the last mile. Do isometric exercises while you are watching a movie or television. Give it some thought. You might be surprised at the number of different ways you can add regular exercise to your everyday activities.

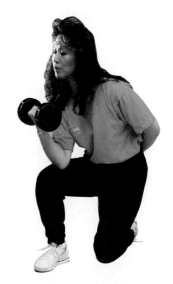

USING WHAT YOU HAVE LEARNED Throughout this book, you have learned a great deal about health and fitness. The 5 *W*'s and 1 *H*, which are listed below, summarize the topics you have been reading about. For a lifetime of fitness, apply what you have learned in the years to come.

- **Who** can become fit.
- **Why** you should exercise, reduce stress, and eat right.
- **What** exercises, sports, and activities you should do and should avoid; and what nutrients you should eat and should avoid.
- **When** you should exercise, relax, and nourish your body.
- **Where** you can or should exercise and relax.
- **How** you should exercise, relax, and eat.

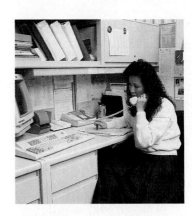

Build regular activity into your daily life.

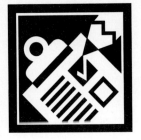

SELF-EVALUATION

ATTITUDES TOWARD FITNESS

WORKSHEET 18-1

Use worksheet 18-1 to reevaluate your attitudes toward fitness.

In Chapter 1, you evaluated your attitudes about exercise and fitness. By now, you have learned a great deal more about fitness and tried many different exercises, activities, and sports. Now take time to reexamine your fitness attitudes.

Use the questionnaire on worksheet 18-1 to evaluate how you feel now about fitness and exercise. Do *not* try to recall how you felt earlier in this course. Just think about how you feel now.

After you have completed your self-evaluation, ask yourself these questions. How has my attitude toward fitness changed? Do I have a more or a less positive attitude now? If you have started to exercise regularly, your attitude has improved—whether or not you were aware of it. If you have not started to exercise regularly, your attitude needs to improve. Think about ways to change your fitness attitude. You can start by trying to determine the reasons why you do not like to exercise. Then, see what you can do to overcome these obstacles.

LIFELONG ATTITUDES

Many people can be categorized according to their attitudes toward fitness. Do you recognize yourself in any of the types below?

- **Wishers** Wishers usually just sit back and wish they were fit and healthy, instead of doing something to improve their fitness.
- **Talkers** These people talk about what they will do to improve their fitness when they have time, but they rarely act on what they say.
- **Pessimists** Pessimistic people often see only the downside of a situation. Often they resort to making fun of people who are slimmer, more fit, or more skilled than they are. They also might criticize exercise programs and equipment. Instead of criticizing, they should act to improve their own health and fitness.
- **Optimists** Optimistic people usually are quick to see the positive aspects of a situation. They recognize the benefits of good health and fitness, and *act* to improve themselves. They stick with their fitness program and goals even when progress is slow, because they do not expect results to come instantly.

HAVE YOU HEARD?

Eula Weaver is an example of an optimist. Several years ago, her doctor told her she must walk regularly to improve her failing cardiovascular system. Now Ms. Weaver jogs a mile each day. She's 87 years old!

CHAPTER REVIEW

MULTIPLE CHOICE
Choose the letter of the best answer.

1. Which is *not* a possible meaning for the term "fitness for life?" (a) A fit person enjoys life more. (b) A person should strive for fitness for his or her entire life. (c) Fit people are more likely to live longer. (d) Fitness is nice, but not needed for survival.

2. Being fit guarantees that you will (a) have a long life. (b) feel and look better. (c) have good health. (d) be stronger than most people your age.

3. Which probably is *least* important for a happy, productive life? (a) good mental health (b) beauty (c) health-related fitness (d) skill-related fitness

4. Which is *not* one of the items recommended to help build fitness self-discipline? (a) create a place to work-out at home (b) join a summer sports or fitness program (c) join a health club (d) increase the amount of activity in your daily life

5. Which person likely has the best attitude about fitness? (a) one who exercises once a week (b) weekend athlete (c) one who exercises regularly (d) one who does not exercise

6. Which is *incorrectly* associated with old age? (a) poor physical fitness (b) gray hair (c) decline in vision (d) decline in hearing

7. Use the *5 W*s and *1 H* to (a) plan an exercise program. (b) describe exercises. (c) explain nutrient needs. (d) summarize fitness topics.

MATCHING
Match the definition in Column I with the term it defines in Column II.

Column I	Column II
8. encourages you in your effort to become fit	a. optimist
9. thinks about exercising, but does not do it	b. pessimist
10. criticizes exercise programs	c. support group
11. exercises regularly even when progress is slow	d. talker
12. talks about exercise, but rarely exercises	e. wisher

FOCUS ON FITNESS

OTHER SPORTS AND ACTIVITIES FOR A LIFETIME

At the end of each chapter in this book, you have read about different sports and activities that you can continue to play for a lifetime. The activities and sports shown here are but a few of dozens of lifetime sports and activities.

Try as many of these or other sports and activities as possible, not because you should do *all* of them, but so that you can find out which ones you enjoy most. Too many people say, "That's not for me," without even trying the activity. The activities you choose do not *all* have to be good for developing fitness. You might want to do some just for fun, but do include some kinds of exercise that will build each of the health-related parts of fitness.

BOWLING

Bowling can help improve parts of skill-related fitness, such as coordination and balance. Points are scored depending upon the number of bowling pins knocked down in each part, or frame, of a game. Instruction can familiarize you with the basics of bowling, though practice is most important for improving skills. Many people bowl in competitive leagues throughout the year.

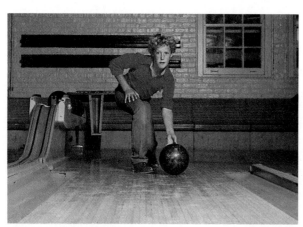

RACQUETBALL

Racquetball is a fast-paced game that can be played with 2, 3, or 4 players. The game is a challenge, both in skill and strategy. The racquetball court is a high-walled room with wood flooring. Players use the side and back walls to hit the ball back to the front wall and score points. A racquetball racquet and racquet balls are the only equipment required, though goggles for eye protection are highly recommended. Many facilities offer lessons and can help schedule matches and tournaments for players.

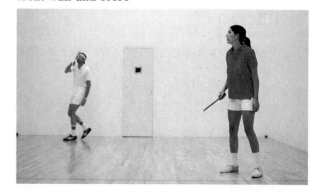

SKIING

Skiing is a sport that all can enjoy. Even handicapped individuals can ski. Downhill skiing and cross-country skiing are the two most popular forms of skiing. Cross-country skiing is particularly good for developing cardiovascular fitness. Basic equipment for both downhill and cross-country skiing can be rented or purchased. Beginning skiers should take lessons, often available through community recreation programs and most ski resorts.

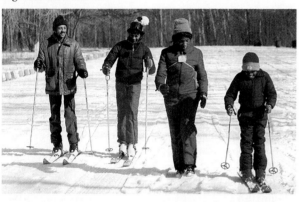

BADMINTON

You can play badminton in your backyard or on an official court. It is played by hitting a "bird" (shuttlecock) with a racquet back and forth across a net to an opponent. As with other sports, many schools and recreation centers sponsor informal badminton leagues and tournaments.

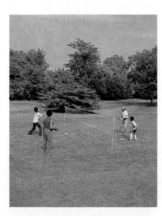

HORSEBACK RIDING

Horseback riding can provide good exercise and is also an enjoyable activity. A great deal of skill is not needed, but proper instruction is recommended. Since owning your own horse and riding equipment can be very expensive, most people rent a horse and equipment to ride.

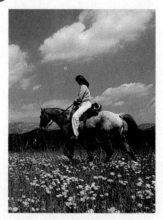

ARCHERY

Archery is one of the most interesting activities available. It requires no partner or team, and is a good family activity because it can be enjoyed by both sexes and all ages. Archery is easily adapted for most handicapped people. Equipment varies depending upon the type of archery chosen. For safety, good equipment and shooting areas are necessary. Most cities have clubs, and many schools conduct classes in archery techniques.

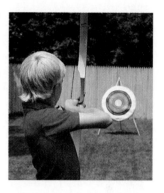

GOLF

Millions of people enjoy golf. The game is a challenge, both in strategy and in skill. No two golf shots are ever the same, and a player always trys to achieve a better score. Public courses and private clubs are available for golf. Most courses have equipment for rent and offer group or private lessons for a fee. Many schools and community centers also offer group lessons.

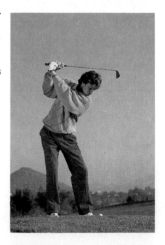

TENNIS

Tennis appeals to people of all ages. Like racquetball, tennis can be played with 2, 3, or 4 players. Most community centers and many schools offer tennis lessons for all levels of ability. Both indoor and outdoor tennis courts are usually available in most communities, making tennis a good year-round sport.

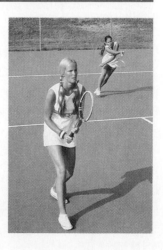

CALORIE VALUES

Bread-Cereal Group

Bagel, 1 165
Biscuit, 1 105
Bun, 1 120
Bread
    raisin, 1 slice 65
    rye, 1 slice 60
    white, 1 slice 65
    whole wheat, 1 slice 60
Cereal
    bran flakes, 1 cup 105
    corn flakes, 1 cup 95
    oatmeal, 1 cup 130
    puffed oats, 1 cup 100
    puffed rice, 1 cup 60
    puffed wheat, 1 cup 55
    shredded wheat, 1 biscuit 55
    wheat flakes, 1 cup 105
Crackers
    graham, 1 55
    saltine, 1 50
Muffin
    blueberry, 1 medium 110
    bran, 1 medium 105
    corn, 1 medium 125
    plain, 1 medium 120
Noodle, egg, 1 cup 200
Pancake, 1 small 60
Popcorn, plain, 1 cup 145
Pretzel, 1 25
Rice, 1 cup 180
Spaghetti, plain, 1 cup 190
Tortilla, corn, 1 70
Waffle, 1 205

Fruit-Vegetable Group

Alfalfa sprouts, 1/2 cup 19
Apple, 1 medium 80
Applesauce, 1 cup 100
Asparagus, 1 spear 25
Avocado, 1 medium 370
Banana, 1 medium 100
Beans
    green, 1 cup 30
    lima, 1 cup 170
    red kidney, 1 cup 230
Broccoli, 1 stalk 10
Cabbage, 1 cup 15
Carrot, 1 medium 30

Cauliflower, 1 cup 30
Celery, 1 stalk 5
Cherries, 1 5
Corn, 1 ear 70
Cucumber, 6 large slices 5
Grapes, green, 1 3
Grapefruit, 1/2 50
Juice
    apple, 1 cup 120
    cranberry, 1 cup 165
    grape, 1 cup 165
    grapefruit, 1 cup 100
    lemonade, 1 cup 105
    orange, 1 cup 120
    pineapple, 1 cup 140
    tomato, 1 cup 45
Lettuce, head, 1 wedge 20
Melon
    cantaloupe, 1/2 80
    honeydew, 1/10 50
    watermelon, 1 wedge 110
Mushrooms, 1 cup 90
Olives
    black, ripe, 2 large 15
    green, 3 extra large 15
Onion, green, 1 3
Orange, 1 medium 65
Peach, 1 medium 40
Pear, 1 medium 100
Peas, green, 1 cup 110
Pineapple, 1 cup 80
Potato, baked, 1 medium 145
Radish, 1 1
Raisins, 1 cup 420
Strawberries, 1 cup 55
Spinach, 1 cup cooked 40
Squash
    summer, 1 cup 30
    winter, 1 cup 130
Sweet pepper, 1 medium 15
Sweet potato, baked, 1 160
Tomato, 1 medium 25

Meat-Poultry-Fish-Bean Group

Bacon, fried, 2 slices 85
Beef
    ground, broiled, 3 oz. 185
    roast, 3 oz. 375
    steak, 3 oz. 330

Chicken
    broiled, ¹/₂ broiler, 10 oz. 240
    fried, breast, 2.8 oz. 160
Egg
    fried, 1 85
    hard-cooked, 1 80
Ham
    baked, 3 oz. 245
    boiled, 1 oz. 65
Lamb, chop, broiled, 3 oz. 360
Pork
    chop, broiled 3 oz. 305
    roast, 3 oz. 310
    with baked beans, 1 cup 310
Salmon, pink, canned 120
Sausage
    bologna, 1 slice 85
    frankfurter, 1 170
Seeds and nuts
    almond, 1 cup 690
    cashew, 1 cup 785
    coconut, 1 cup 275
    peanut, 1 cup 840
    pecan, 1 cup 810
    pumpkin, 1 cup 775
    sunflower, 1 cup 810
Shrimp, fried, 3 oz. 190
Tuna, canned in oil, 3 oz. 170

Milk Group

Butter, 1 tbsp. 100
Cheese
    American, 1 oz. 100
    cheddar, 1 oz. 105
    cottage
        creamed, 1 cup 235
        low-fat, 1 cup 125
    cream, 1 oz. 100
    Swiss, 1 oz. 95
Cream
    half and half, 1 tbsp. 20
    sour, 1 tbsp. 25
    whipped, 1 tbsp. 80
Milk
    low-fat 1%, 1 cup 120
    low-fat 2%, 1 cup 150
    skim, 1 cup 85
    whole, 1 cup 165
Yogurt, low-fat, 1 cup 145

Other Foods

Beverages
    soft drink, 12 oz. 145
    diet soft drink, 12 oz. 1
Cake
    angel food, ¹/₁₂ 135
    cupcake, no icing, 1 90
    chocolate, iced, ¹/₁₂ 235
Candy
    milk chocolate, 1 oz. 145
    hard, 1 oz. 110
Catsup, 1 tbsp. 17
Cookies
    brownie, 1 small 95
    chocolate chip, 1 small 50
    oatmeal/raisin 60
    chocolate sandwich, 1 50
Doughnut, plain, 1 100
Gelatin, flavored, 1 cup 140
Honey, 1 tbsp. 65
Ice cream
    regular, 1 cup 140
    sherbet, 1 cup 270
Jam, 1 tbsp. 55
Jelly, 1 tbsp. 50
Margarine, 1 tbsp. 50
Mayonnaise, 1 tbsp. 100
Mustard, 1 tsp. 5
Oil
    corn, 1 tbsp. 120
    olive, 1 tbsp. 120
    peanut, 1 tbsp. 120
    safflower, 1 tbsp. 120
Peanut butter, 1 tbsp. 95
Pickles
    dill, 1 medium 5
    sweet, 1 small 20
Pie
    apple, ¹/₈ pie 345
    cherry, ¹/₈ pie 350
    lemon meringue, ¹/₈ pie 305
Potato chips, 10 115
Salad dressing
    French, 1 tbsp. 65
    Italian, 1 tbsp. 85
    thousand island, 1 tbsp. 80
Sugar, granulated, 1 tbsp. 45
Table syrup, 1 tbsp. 60

CALORIE VALUES (FAST FOODS)

Burger King
Cheeseburger, 1 305
French fries, 1 regular order 315
Hamburger, 1 250
Vanilla shake, 1 330
Whaler® 585
Whopper®, 1 660

Dairy Queen
Big Braiser® Deluxe, 1 470
Big Braiser® Regular, 1 460
Braiser® dog, 1 275
Braiser® French fries, 1 regular order 320
Braiser® onion rings, 1 order 300
Fish sandwich, 1 400

Dunkin' Donuts
Blueberry muffin, 1 280
Bran muffin, 1 320
Coffee roll, honey-dipped, 1 330
Donut
   plain cake, 1 275
   raised, honey-dipped, 1 225
Munch-kins®
   plain cake, 1 50
   raised, honey-dipped, 1 35

Kentucky Fried Chicken
Individual pieces (Original Recipe®)
   breast, 1 240
   drumstick, 1 135
   thigh, 1 275
   wing, 1 150

Long John Silver's
Chicken Planks®, 4 pieces 460
Cole slaw, 4 oz. 140
Corn on the cob, 1 175
Fish with batter, 2 pieces 320
French fries, 3 oz. 320
Hush puppies, 3 155
Shrimp with batter, 6 pieces 270

McDonald's
Big Mac®, 1 560
Cheeseburger, 1 310
Egg McMuffin®, 1 290
Filet O'Fish®, 1 440
French fries, 1 regular order 305
Hamburger, 1 260
Hot cakes, with butter and syrup 410
Salad
   chef, plain, 1 225
   chicken oriental, plain, 1 140
   garden, plain, 1 110
Salad dressing
   blue cheese, 1 package 340
   house, 1 package 325
   oriental, 1 package 100
   thousand island, 1 package 390
Scrambled eggs, 1 serving 140
Quarter Pounder®, 1 410

Pizza Hut
(*Note:* 1 serving equals $\frac{1}{2}$ of a 10-inch pizza.)
Thick 'n' Chewy®
   cheese, 1 serving 560
   pepperoni, 1 serving 560
   supreme, 1 serving 640
Thin 'n' Crispy®
   cheese, 1 serving 450
   pepperoni, 1 serving 430
   supreme, 1 serving 510

Taco Bell
Bean burrito, 1 345
Beef burrito, 1 465
Beefy tostada, 1 290
Burrito supreme, 1 460
Combination burrito, 1 405
Pintos 'n' Cheese, 1 170
Taco, 1 185
Tostada, 1 180

Target Body Weight: Females (age 14–18)

Actual Body Weight	Sum of Triceps and Calf Skinfolds									
	27–28	29–30	31–32	33–35	36–38	39–42	43–45	47–49	50–52	53+
200	197	193	189	185	181	177	173	169	165	161
195	192	188	184	180	176	172	168	164	160	157
190	187	183	179	175	172	168	164	160	156	153
185	182	178	174	171	167	163	160	156	152	149
180	177	173	170	166	163	159	155	152	148	145
175	172	169	165	162	158	155	151	148	144	141
170	167	164	160	157	154	150	147	143	140	137
165	162	159	156	151	149	146	142	139	136	133
160	157	154	151	148	145	141	138	135	132	129
155	152	149	146	143	140	137	134	131	128	125
150	148	145	142	139	136	133	130	127	124	121
145	143	140	137	134	131	128	125	122	119	117
140	138	135	132	129	127	124	121	118	115	114
135	133	130	127	125	122	119	117	114	111	109
130	128	125	123	120	118	115	112	110	107	105
125	123	121	118	116	113	111	108	106	103	101
120	118	116	113	111	109	106	104	101	99	97
115	113	111	109	106	104	102	99	97	95	93
110	108	106	104	102	100	97	95	93	91	89
105	103	101	99	97	95	93	91	89	87	85
100	99	97	95	93	91	89	87	85	83	81
95	94	92	90	88	86	84	82	80	78	77
90	89	87	85	83	82	80	78	76	74	73
85	84	82	80	78	77	75	72	70	68	67

Target Body Weight: Males (age 14–18)

Actual Body Weight	Sum of Triceps and Calf Skinfolds									
	22–23	24–25	26–28	29–31	32–34	35–37	38–40	41–42	43–45	46+
240	234	230	225	220	215	210	206	201	196	191
235	229	225	220	215	210	206	201	196	192	187
230	224	220	215	210	206	201	197	192	187	183
225	220	216	211	207	202	198	193	189	184	180
220	215	211	206	202	197	193	189	184	180	175
215	210	206	201	197	193	188	184	180	175	171
210	205	202	200	192	188	184	180	175	171	167
205	200	197	191	187	183	179	175	171	167	163
200	196	192	188	184	180	176	172	168	164	160
195	190	187	183	179	175	171	167	163	159	155
190	185	182	178	174	170	166	163	159	155	151
185	180	177	173	169	165	162	158	154	151	147
180	175	172	168	164	161	157	154	150	146	143
175	171	168	164	161	157	154	150	147	143	140
170	166	163	159	156	152	149	146	142	139	135
165	161	158	154	151	148	144	141	138	134	131
160	157	153	149	146	143	140	137	133	130	127
155	151	148	144	141	138	135	132	129	126	123
150	147	144	141	138	135	132	129	126	123	120
145	141	139	136	133	130	127	124	121	118	115
140	136	134	131	128	125	122	120	117	114	111
135	131	129	126	123	120	118	115	112	110	107
130	126	124	121	118	116	113	111	108	105	103
125	122	120	117	115	112	110	107	105	102	100
120	117	115	112	110	107	105	103	100	98	95

CAREERS

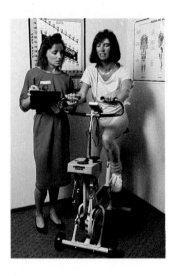

ATHLETIC TRAINER

Professional athletes follow carefully planned training programs to stay fit. However, even with this training, athletes sometimes suffer injuries. Athletic trainers work with athletes to help them recover from injuries.

Many athletic trainers work for a particular school or college athletic department. Still others work for professional sports teams. Trainers travel with the team, attend team functions and games, and are prepared to give medical aid when an athlete is injured. Athletes with serious injuries are referred to medical doctors. Athletic trainers also oversee recovery programs for injured athletes, and keep track of the general health of all athletes.

Most athletic trainers attend at least four years of college. Many receive training in professions such as physical therapy or nursing. Many continue their studies, complete an internship, and pass an examination to become certified athletic trainers. For more information, write:

National Athletic Trainers Association
2952 Stemmons Freeway
Dallas, TX   75247

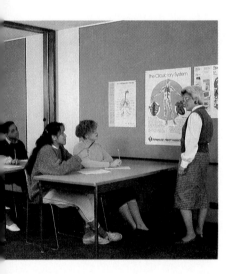

HEALTH EDUCATOR

Health educators work in all aspects of health and health problems. They work to inform the public, through schools and other locations, about current health-related findings. They conduct surveys to determine how well people are informed about current health problems.

Some health educators direct community health programs. They work to raise community interest in such areas as alcohol and drug abuse, chronic disease, and environmental issues. Health educators often speak to health-care professionals and community organizations. They use the media to make the public aware of available health programs.

Public health educators have four-year degrees in health or community health education. Many jobs also require a master's degree. For more information, write:

Association for the Advancement of Health Education
1900 Association Drive
Reston, VA 22091

PHYSICAL EDUCATION TEACHER

Physical education teachers play an important role in the physical well-being of individuals of all ages. They recognize that good physical education programs increase the general health of the participants. They design programs to meet that need. Physical education teachers know that these programs educate people to think logically and accurately and how to use these skills throughout their lives. Good physical education programs also help people mature emotionally, as well as physically, so they are better able to handle stressful situations.

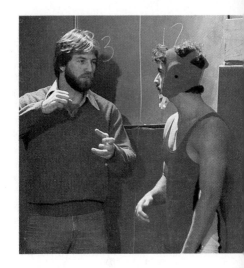

Physical education teachers work in elementary schools, high schools, and colleges. Some physical educators coach in addition to teaching. However, some are employed by community recreation centers. Career opportunities are increasing in industries that sponsor employee fitness programs and centers.

Most teachers have four-year or six-year degrees in physical education from a university or college. For more information, write:
Alliance for Health, Physical Education, Recreation, and Dance
1900 Association Drive
Reston, VA 22091

PHYSICAL THERAPIST

Physical therapists work with people who have handicaps resulting from a variety of causes, including diseases, inherited disorders, and accidents. A physical therapist studies a patient's case to determine what short-term and long-term goals are possible. The physical therapist uses heat, cold, massage, exercise, electricity, ultrasonic devices, and other sophisticated techniques to strengthen and stimulate a patient's muscles. The goal is to help a patient to regain as much movement as possible, considering their condition.

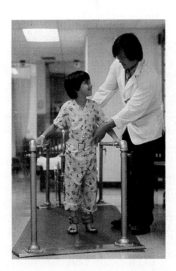

Most physical therapists work in health clinics, hospitals, and nursing homes. Some work with one or more doctors on a consulting basis. Following a four-year degree in physical therapy, a physical therapist must have at least four months of experience in a health-care facility working with a licensed therapist. All states require physical therapists to be licensed. For more information, write:
American Physical Therapy Association
1111 North Fairfax Street
Alexandria, VA 22314

GLOSSARY

A

activity neurosis, being overly concerned about getting enough exercise

aerobic dance, a combination of dance steps and calisthenics done to music

aerobic exercise, steady exercise in which the heart can supply all the oxygen your muscles need

agility, ability to change the position of your body quickly and to control your body's movements

amino acids, the building blocks of proteins

anabolic steroid, a dangerous substance that makes muscles more bulky but can cause bodily harm

anaerobic exercise, exercise done in short, fast bursts in which the heart cannot supply blood and oxygen as fast as muscles use it

anorexia nervosa, an eating disorder in which a person severely limits food intake

artery, a blood vessel that carries blood from your heart to other parts of your body

atherosclerosis, a disease in which the arteries become dangerously clogged with deposits

B

balance, ability to keep an upright posture while standing still or moving

ballistic stretching, a series of quick but gentle bouncing or bobbing motions that are not held for a long time

biomechanical principle, a rule that helps the human machine work and play efficiently

blood pressure, the force with which blood pushes against artery walls

body fatness, percentage of body weight that is fat

bulimia, a pattern of overeating followed by forced vomiting or use of laxatives to rid the body of food

C

calipers, a tool to measure skinfold

calisthenics, exercises done using your body weight as resistance

Calorie, a heat unit that refers to the energy available in food

carbohydrates, nutrients, especially sugars and starches, that furnish energy

cardiac muscle, a type of muscle that makes up the heart

cardiovascular fitness, ability to exercise for long periods of time because you have a strong heart, healthy lungs, and clear blood vessels

cardiovascular system, the heart and blood vessels, the body system that moves oxygen and nutrients to body cells and removes cell wastes

cholesterol, a fat-like substance found in animal cells and in some foods, such as dairy products and egg yolks

complex carbohydrates, nutrients, mainly starches and fibers, made of long chains of simple sugars

controllable risk factor, a risk factor that you can act upon to change

cool-down, the last stage of an exercise program, consisting of exercises to help return heart rate to normal and to prevent muscle soreness

coordination, ability to use your senses together with your body parts or to use two or more body parts together

D

dehydrated, lacking normal amount of body fluid

diastolic blood pressure, the lowest blood pressure exerted by the blood within your arteries

diet, a person's eating habits

distress, situations that produce "bad" stress

E

essential amino acids, eight amino acids the body cannot manufacture and must obtain through food

essential body fat, the minimum amount of body fat that a person should possess

eustress, situations that produce "good" stress

F

fad diet, a nutritionally unbalanced diet that falsely promises a quick weight loss

fast-twitch red muscle fibers, muscle fibers that contract at a fast rate and have strength as well as endurance

fast-twitch white muscle fibers, muscle fibers that contract at a fast rate and have great strength but very little endurance

fats, nutrients that provide energy, help growth and repair of cells, and dissolve and carry certain vitamins to cells

fiber, a type of indigestible carbohydrate

FIT formula, consists of three factors in all fitness programs: frequency, intensity, and time

flexibility, ability to use your joints fully through a wide range of motion

food supplement, a product intended to add nutrients to a person's diet

four food groups, include the meat-poultry-fish-bean group, the bread-cereal group, the fruit-vegetable group, and the milk group

frequency, how often a person exercises

frostbite, damage to body tissue caused by cold

H

health-related fitness, the parts of physical fitness that include cardiovascular fitness, strength, muscular endurance, flexibility, body fatness

heart attack, condition resulting from severely reduced blood supply to the heart muscle

heart cool-down, a slow-moving activity to help your heart and blood vessels return to normal after vigorous exercise

heart rate, the number of times your heart beats per minute

heart warm-up, several minutes of slow exercise that gradually increases the heart rate for more vigorous exercise

heat exhaustion, condition caused by excessive exposure to heat, characterized by cold, clammy skin and symptoms of shock

heat stroke, condition caused by exposure to excessive heat, characterized by high fever and dry skin

heredity, the passing of genetic traits from parents to children

high-density lipoproteins (HDL), often referred to as "good cholesterol" because HDLs carry excess cholesterol out of the bloodstream

high-intensity exercise, can build muscular endurance needed for high-level performance

hyperkinetic condition, condition caused by doing too much exercise

hypertension, condition in which the blood pressure is consistently higher than normal

hyperventilate, breathe too quickly

hypokinetic condition, a health problem associated with, or caused by, a lack of physical activity or regular exercise

hypothermia, a lowering of body temperature usually caused by excessive exposure to cold

I

incomplete proteins, foods that contain some of, but not all, the essential amino acids

insomnia, difficulty getting to sleep and staying asleep

intensity, how hard a person exercises

intermediate fibers, muscle fibers that have characteristics of both slow- and fast-twitch fibers

interval training, anaerobic exercise in which fast movements over a short distance alternate with slower exercise

involuntary muscles, smooth and cardiac muscles, the contractions of which you cannot consciously control

isometric exercise, exercise in which the muscles contract when working against a stationary object but body parts do not move

isotonic exercise, exercise in which muscles contract and move parts of the body

J

joint, place in the body where bones come together

L

ligament, tough, white tissue that connects bones

lordosis, swayback, an abnormal curve of the spine

low-density lipoproteins (LDL), often referred to as "bad cholesterol" because LDLs carry cholesterol that might stay in the body

low-impact aerobics, aerobic exercise in which one foot contacts the floor at all times

low-intensity exercise, level of exercise that builds muscular endurance needed for daily activities

M

medium-intensity exercise, the level of exercise that builds muscular endurance needed for doing vigorous activities without tiring quickly

microtrauma, an injury, often caused by harmful exercise, that produces pain or soreness long after the injury occurs, but not immediately

minerals, nutrients that perform many functions in regulating the activities of cells

muscle-bound, a condition in which tight, bulky muscles prevent free movement

muscle cool-down and stretch, a stage of exercising that helps prevent muscle soreness by slowly stretching muscles used in a workout

muscle cramp, a spasm or sudden tightening of a muscle

muscle warm-up and stretch, mild exercises that gently stretch and help contract your muscles in preparation for a workout

muscular endurance, ability to use your muscles many times without tiring

N

noncontrollable risk factor, a risk factor that you cannot change

nutrients, food substances required for the growth and maintenance of cells

nutrition, the study of foods and how they nourish the body

nutritionally dense, describes foods that contain large amounts of nutrients for the number of Calories provided

O

obesity, having a high percentage of body fat

orienteering, a combination of walking, jogging, and map reading

osteoporosis, a condition in which the bones become porous and start to lose their strength

overload, *see:* principle of overload

overuse injury, damage to bones, muscles, or other tissues by excessive exercise

P

parcourse, an outdoor course containing exercise stations with signs suggesting the number of *Physical Activity Repetitions* for each exercise.

passive exercise, ineffective exercises that do not stretch muscles nor make them contract

perception, how you interpret a situation

physical fitness, ability of body systems to work together efficiently

power, ability to use strength quickly

principle of overload, improving fitness by doing more exercise than you usually do

principle of progression, a gradual increase in exercise as to stay within your target fitness zone

principle of specificity, doing specific activities to build specific parts of fitness

protein, nutrients that build and repair your body cells

psychological stressors, or mental stressors, are caused by your own feelings

Q

quackery, advertising or selling of worthless services and products

R

reaction time, amount of time it takes you to move once you realize the need to act

registered dietitian, a person qualified to give advice about food and diet

rehydrated, drinking liquids to replace those lost through exercise or other activity

repetitions, the number of consecutive times you do each exercise

respiratory system, the body system that includes your lungs, brings oxygen to your bloodstream, and eliminates carbon dioxide from your bloodstream

resting heart rate, the number of heartbeats when you are relatively inactive

risk factor, anything that increases your chance of something occurring

runner's heel, a soreness in the heel usually caused by running or jumping activities in which the heel hits the ground repeatedly

S

saturated fat, a nutrient found in dairy products and animal fat

set, a group of repetitions

shin splint, a soreness in the front of the lower leg probably caused by small muscle tears or muscle spasms from overuse of the muscle

side stitch, a pain in the side of the lower abdomen that a person might experience while exercising

simple carbohydrates, sugars that can be used by your body with little or no change during digestion

skeletal muscle, muscle attached to bones that makes movement possible

skill-related fitness, basic abilities that help you learn particular skills

skinfold, fold of skin and underlying fat which, when measured with calipers, indicate the percentage of body fat

slow-twitch muscle fibers, muscle that contracts at a slow rate and has great endurance

smooth muscle, muscle that makes up the walls of hollow internal organs such as the stomach and blood vessels

speed, ability to perform a movement or cover a distance in a short period of time

speedplay, an activity that includes walking, jogging, calisthenics, and sprints

sprain, an injury to ligaments and muscles

static stretching, stretching slowly as far as you can and then holding the stretch for several seconds

strain, an injury to a tendon or muscle

strength, amount of force your muscles can produce

stress, the body's reaction to a demanding situation

stressor, anything that causes or contributes to stress

stress response, the "fight or flight" response

stress test, a measure of how your heart responds to vigorous exercise

stroke, loss of some of a person's abilities due to a broken or blocked blood vessel in the brain

systolic blood pressure, the highest pressure exerted by blood within your arteries

T

target ceiling, the upper limit of your target fitness zone

target fitness zone, the right amount of exercise to build your fitness

target weight, ideal weight, the weight at which you have the proper amount of body fat

threshold of training, the minimum amount of overload necessary to build physical fitness

time, how long a person exercises

total fitness, fitness of the whole person including, physical, mental, social, and emotional fitness

U

underfat, having too little body fat

unsaturated fat, nutrient found in many oils, such as olive oil and peanut oil

V

vein, a blood vessel that carries blood to the heart

vitamins, nutrients needed for growth and repair of body cells

voluntary muscle, skeletal muscle, muscle the activity of which you can control

W

warm-up, first stage of an exercise program, usually consisting of a muscle warm-up and stretch and a heart warm-up

workout, the second stage, or vigorous part, of your exercise program

INDEX

ACKNOWLEDGMENTS

PHOTOGRAPHS

Unless otherwise acknowledged, all photographs are the property of Scott, Foresman and Company. The abbreviations indicate position of pictures: (t)top, (b)bottom, (l)left, (r)right, (c)center.

Page 46: National Heart, Lung, and Blood Institute, National Institutes of Health. **90:** Courtesy, Universal Gym Equipment, Inc., Cedar Rapids, Iowa. **180:** National Council Against Health Fraud, Inc. **198:** ©Mickey Pfleger. **210:** (r), David Madison. **221:** (tl), Brent Jones; (bl), Rob Brown/Focus on Sports; (cr), ALL SPORT USA. **226:** (t), Brian Drake/Sportschrome. **227:** (t), David Madison.

TEXT

Page 59: From THE NEW AEROBICS by Kenneth H. Cooper. Copyright © 1970 by Kenneth H. Cooper. Reprinted by permission of Bantam Books, a division of Bantam, Doubleday, Dell Publishing Group, Inc. **74:** Aerobic dance routine choreographed by Rita Oechsner. **127:** "Triceps Plus Calf Skinfolds: Males" and "Triceps Plus Calf Skinfolds: Females" reprinted by permission of Dr. Tim G. Lohman, Department of Exercise and Sport Sciences, University of Arizona. **128:** "Body Measurement: Males" and "Body Measurement: Females" by Jack Wilmore. Reprinted by permission of the author.